BODY TRANSFORMATION

LOSE WEIGHT,
GAIN ENERGY
&
REVERSE PREMATURE AGING

JULIE CHRYSTYN

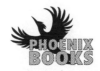

PHOENIX BOOKS

The information contained in this book is based upon the research and personal experiences of the author. This information is not intended as a substitute for consulting with your physician or other health care provider. The publisher and the author are not responsible for any adverse effects or consequences resulting from the use of any of the suggestions, preparations, or procedures in this book. All matters pertaining to your diet, exercise and physical health should be supervised by a health care professional.

ISBN: 1-59777-521-5

Library of Congress Cataloging-In-Publication Data Available

Book Design by: Sonia Fiore

Printed in the United States of America

Phoenix Books
9465 Wilshire Boulevard, Suite 315
Beverly Hills, CA 90212

10 9 8 7 6 5 4 3 2 1

TO

TAYLOR ROSE

ACKNOWLEDGEMENTS

B *ody Transformation* would not have happened without the encouragement of the late Diana, Princess of Wales. She eagerly chose to offer her public endorsement of the original, pre-updated version of this book, which would have made it her first, and perhaps only, gesture of its kind. The Princess would have followed the lead of Dr. Ronald Davey, The Queen's personal physician of many years, who during his long and distinguished career gave his only commercial book endorsement to my previous health book, *Life Force*, a number of years earlier. The Princess developed a passion for healthy living as she made many efforts to help herself cope with the physical and emotional pain and strain of her complicated life. She was eager to share what she learned and to help others—this was no exception. Hence, with or without her influence at present, now as then, I offer my heartfelt gratitude to the late Princess Diana.

After her untimely death, I placed this book on the shelf. Nevertheless, I thank the wonderful people at Bantam Books for making the first purchase, as well as Random House, Penguin and others for their very generous offers. At the end of the day, I chose maverick publisher and media genius

Michael A. Viner. On a daily basis, I am inspired by his example and determination to combat adversity, and to pursue and live for a greater cause. For this, above all, he will always have my utmost respect and admiration.

The one who inspired me first and foremost, however, and taught me the most about healthy living—by example of his very *unhealthy* living—was a human torpedo known as my father. I have learned after his three heart attacks, two strokes, a leg amputation, arterial transplants, an adrenal tumor, type-II diabetes, multiple skin grafts for third-degree burns, prostate surgery, and a smorgasbord of transplants, implants, house plants, and chronic pain that could only be somewhat alleviated with heavy duty prescription narcotics…that a little prevention indeed does go a long way. A year ago last Father's Day, at the age of 64, his body finally gave out after more than six crucifying years following an accident, and $2.7 million in health care costs. I dare say that virtually all of his devastating conditions and unimaginable suffering was preventable and thus self-inflicted. As is always the case, his pain and suffering wasn't only his own; it impacted the lives of everyone else around him. Thus, my objective is to spread the message that _we can do better._

In due time, along came Kenin M. Spivak. The likelihood of convincing this genius mega-executive and living saint to become my manager was about the same as winning the big one in the Lotto. Fortunately, he must have had a karmic debt on his hands, for I won the jackpot. Kenin has enjoyed a distinguished career that combines top-tier success in management, marketing, finance, and law with stints as an investment banker at Merrill Lynch, CEO of a NewsCorp company, COO of MGM/UA, and

CEO of Telemac, among others. Most recently, I thoroughly enjoyed our collaboration on the killer thriller, *The Karasik Conspiracy*. Now, if I can only get him and Mr. Viner to eat better....

My own transformation of a different kind occurred when my priorities shifted thanks to Suzanne von Liebig. She came out of nowhere and rocked my world. Her influence and horse sense has changed me forever.

HRH Princess Elizabeth of Yugoslavia. I'm a native of Croatia who was granted political asylum in the United States around the age of seven. But there's nothing opposite about this union. She is a voice of reason, wisdom, intellect, compassion, and wicked humor. I am forever grateful for her kindness and friendship.

I thank the extraordinary people at Phoenix Books in Beverly Hills for all of their efforts on my behalf, especially Sonia Fiore, Rochelle O'Gorman, Julie McCarron, Sal Preciado and Melody Storm. I am most grateful to the hardest working multitasker anywhere, the diligent and perpetually astute Francine Uyetake, vice-president of Spivak Management, Inc. I also thank SMI's Phil Oster and Stacie Amezuca. And, in a world of great legal minds, few can compare to our much appreciated Ed Lasman.

To a select group of individuals who intentionally and unintentionally influenced the course of my destiny, especially during the four-year production of this book, I offer my most sincere *thank you:* Nely Galan, Marilyn Tam, Dr. Stephen Gullo, John Mappin, Robert Smith, Nabila Khashoggi, Spartan

Daggenhurst, Peter Dekom, Mr. and Mrs. Gerald Cafesjian, Mr. and Mrs. Pierre Falcone, Sherry Antolic, Ana Skoko, Dr. Kathryn Richert-Boe, and Dr. Mel Bottner. Ann Graham, I want to be just like you when I grow up.

I save the most deserving for last, the greatest brother a girl ever had—George Stankovich.

CONTENTS

Part I

Chapter 1   WHAT YOU DON'T KNOW CAN HURT YOU

Chapter 2   ATTITUDE TRANSFORMATION

Chapter 3   MIND TRANSFORMATION

Chapter 4   THE BODY TRANSFORMATION FOOD
             GUIDE PYRAMID

Chapter 5   ARE YOU GOING TO EAT THAT?

Chapter 6   USE IT OR LOSE IT

Part II

Chapter 7   DIGESTION TRANSFORMATION

Chapter 8   IMMUNE FUNCTION TRANSFORMATION

Chapter 9   THE ACID-ALKALINE BALANCE

Chapter 10   ENERGY TRANSFORMATION

Chapter 11   ENDURANCE, STRENGTH AND
             FLEXIBILITY TRANSFORMATION

Chapter 12   HOW TO MAINTAIN YOUR
             BODY TRANSFORMATION

"My people are destroyed for lack of knowledge."

Hosea 4:6

INTRODUCTION

Body Transformation is designed to be your very last diet. Not a "fad diet," but a diet of the right food choices that will make any future dieting for purposes of weight loss, optimum health and longevity virtually obsolete.

Like fads of fashion and style, food fads come and go. There is always a diet trend or craze that's directly related to our desire for weight-loss. But there is nothing faddish about maintaining our proper weight and well-being. Upon closer inspection, fad diets are the same diet plans that are recycled year after year under a new name and fresh marketing campaign. Ultimate weight-loss is always the promise. A magical food is usually identified, a line of miracle-working products generally accompany the books of the more famous diet book authors, and you—the overweight and unhappy individual, is always their target. And their victim. Fad diets are unsuccessful because they violate almost every single principle of healthy eating.

Fortunately, food fads are short-lived. Unfortunately, they perpetually spring up as a *new* fad. For instance, the cabbage soup diet promises a weight loss of 10-17 pounds in just one week of eating nothing but cabbage soup. This is possible, but you would lose that weight primarily due to water loss in your body and the extreme reduction of calories. In the real world, how long do you think you can last eating just one food for a week? And what happens when you resume your regular eating habits? Most people not only regain the weight they starved themselves to lose, but then some!

It cannot be overstated: Dieting is dangerous because it often deprives the body of the nutrients it needs to function properly.

Not so long ago, being overweight was generally seen as a cosmetic problem. We dieted to look better, especially during bathing suit season. We restricted our food intake, eliminated entire food groups, consumed unnatural food preparations, worked-out to the point of exhaustion, and when desperate, paid expensive visits to diet doctors who popularized fad diets and preyed on our vanity.

During the last decade, however, medical science has come to the conclusion that being overweight, especially obese, is public health enemy #1. Today, government statistics list overweight as the leading cause of *preventable* death in the United States.

In our food-saturated environment, for many people losing weight is not a matter of vanity, but survival. For the rest of us—more than half the U.S. population, losing weight is a matter of having greater energy, vitality, and abundant health, to be free of disease. At the same time, vanity gets a nod as we not only feel better, but look better as well.

There are no healthy short cuts to losing weight, but there are smart food choices that will naturally cause weight loss and help you maintain your ideal weight. Today, we are so removed from real food that most people don't even know what we should and shouldn't eat. Thus, we fall prey to popular diets with their contradicting advice that even the most touted experts can't seem to agree on. At the end of the day, we have only succeeded in perpetuating our dangerous weight and health issues.

The bottom line is that the food you eat will either help to destroy or extend your life. Simultaneously, it will determine not only the quantity but quality of your life. A happy, healthy, and long life is less in your genes than in your actions.

Body Transformation is about life-long smart food choices. It is not a short-term diet plan. However, you will begin to see and feel results almost immediately. Once you start to feel good, alert, and happy, you simply won't want to return to your old way of eating. At first glance, you may wonder about the expense of eating this well or the convenient availability of the foods you need. But upon closer examination, these foods are far more economical than the prepackaged and fast foods that you are buying now. You will also find that once you know what to look for, it is far more available that you previously thought. Yes, you are required to do planned shopping and some advance planning, but is your health, happiness, appearance, and well being worth the effort? The time and money it will take for you to transform and maintain your fit and healthy body is merely a fraction of what it would take and cost for you *not* to do it! Remember, you are not only eating for pleasure, you are eating to live and live abundantly.

PART I

CHAPTER 1
WHAT YOU DON'T KNOW
CAN HURT YOU

Optimum health and high energy are the most prized possessions of our time. Consistently, the former and present U.S. Secretary of Health and Human Services state that, "Health is the #1 status symbol" of the new millennium. How is it then that our most precious natural resource is in such scarce supply today?

One out of every two people die from heart disease; one out of four people die of cancer. In fact, 90% of our population is said to be in a pre-cancerous state. The vast majority of our visits to doctors are for complaints about exhaustion, chronic fatigue and other *stress*-related conditions—the precursors to illness.

While economic prosperity and the Information Age is enabling us to be at our best, so many of us are at our personal worst. More money and greater availability has *not* brought us better quality food or healthier bodies. At the same time, greater access to health and diet information simultaneously means an overabundance of *mis*-information.

We are so anxious to lose weight that there is currently a virtual black-out concerning what the trendy new diets are doing to our health and longevity. The truth about what nourishes and sustains life seems to have gone the way of the dinosaur and the Dodo bird.

Needless to say, the trend set by the media is to be thin, thinner, thinnest, emaciated, probably terminal, and possibly the reanimated living dead. A sane person's first question would be: Why look sickly or worse, like you are dying? How can that concentration camp look be so popular today at one extreme, while so much of the population is not just overweight, but morbidly obese?

Our celebrity consumed culture today has a lot to do with it. The media's obsessive and schizophrenic coverage of every star that has gained or lost weight instantly makes her worthy of front page coverage for virtually every weekly celebrity publication, not to mention the dizzying array of celebrity "news" television programs. It would appear that you could become even more famous and further build on a career just by becoming rail thin—it's the fastest way to the spotlight. Just ask Nicole Richie, Lindsay Lohan, Jessica Simpson, and now Kate Hudson, to name but a few.

Let's take a closer look at this phenomenon. Depending on the time of day

We diet in the belief that just about any diet will improve our appearance and health.

and mood of the editor, a star is either "terrifyingly skeletal" or "fitness conscious," while on the treadmill of fame. On June 6, 2005 Lindsay Lohan was "an alarming 112 lbs." according to *Star* magazine. On June 27th, *People* said she was "fitness conscious." On the same June 27th, *Star* called her "terrifyingly skeletal." On July 4th, *In Touch* dubbed her, "gorgeous." But in the same issue, another item said she was "suddenly gaunt." That same July 4th, *Star* said she was "impossibly svelte." On July 11th, *Us Weekly* found her to be "newly chiseled." On the same date, *In Touch* had a revelation for now she was, "shockingly frail."

Nicole Richie's seemingly simple life became increasingly stressful according to her father when the pressures of being in show business overwhelmed her a bit. Once her role on the reality show was over and done with, she remained in the public eye thanks to her shrinking self. On June 13th, *Us Weekly* posed the question, "Too thin?" On June 20th, *Star* replied with, "Super-thin." *Us Weekly* had a comeback on June 20th, "Increasingly unltraskinny." Then *In Touch* jumped into the mix on July 4th, "Gorgeous as the flowers." *People* contributed to the dialogue on July 18th, "You can see her clavicle!" *Us Weekly* rebutted with, "Dazzling." But *In Touch* wasn't going to take it lying down and they fired back with, "almost boyish."

Jessica Simpson with her array of smashing talents got even more attention when she prepared to become a movie star with her role of Daisy Duke, something she "was born to do." On June 6th, *Star* called it as they saw it, "Looking sexy, and flaunting it." Same date, *In Touch* jumped right in with, "Slim...and sexier than ever." Not to be outdone, also on the very same date, *Us Weekly* screamed with a headline, "Brazen sexpot." But Star shot back on June 13th, "A buff, lean and sexy

...we are

sacrificing our

health in order

to meet the

difficult

standard

promoted by

the diet/

beauty/

medical

industry.

body." Wow! Who is her publicist? But then they turned on her. "Denies she's anorexic," *In Touch* reported on June 27th. They went on to say, "Danger Sign: Her ribs are protruding." Two week later, they further saw the light, "Her voluptuous shape has vanished."

Perhaps the working actresses were feeling left out and needed to do something about it. At an airport in Mexico City in 2005, a slumped-over stick figure that looked like a sick homeless person wearing jeans, an oversized T-shirt, and long stringy hair under a hat was on the front page of *The National Enquirer*. Upon closer inspection, it was none other than Kate Hudson. The headline screamed, "Celebrity Deadly Diets."

Sandwiched between Kate and a skeletal Vanessa Paradis (Mrs. Johnny Depp) was a picture of someone's enormous behind with a caption that read, "Guess who? It's not Oprah." Turns out it's Janet Jackson. But not to worry, she'll get serious mileage out of the weight issue once she sheds the pounds and is praised for her newly svelte figure—again.

Take your pick, Hilary Duff, Marcia Cross, Teri Hatcher, Christina Ricci, Alicia Silverstone, Nicole Kidman, and since her divorce, even the already super-fit Jennifer Aniston reportedly went from her thin 120-pounds to an astonishing 112. The past-their-prime stars like Bette Midler, Barbra Streisand and Cybill Shepard are feeling the pressure as well with their weight.

Pick your own shows and movies to watch or models to glance at. No matter where you turn, the vast majority of the females featured in the media are very thin. The powers that profit apparently think that anorexia, bulimia and the drug abuse that's involved in order to achieve this level of thinness is a great way to achieve publicity. In some cases, this is further extended to diet products and books that promote weight-loss but not well-being.

We appear to have no choice but to go on a diet. Preferably the diets that work so well for the stars. Or so we think. However, what many celebrities state in public is not what they do in private. A famous fitness trainer and former model talks about nearly losing her life to anorexia and bulimia while selling the world on her fitness plan. She says that most models follow the ABC Diet: Anorexia, Bulimia, Coffee, Cigarettes, and Cocaine. Kate Moss is the latest casualty at the time of this writing. Perhaps if more companies who hire such models respond as Chanel, Burberry, Christian Dior, and others did in Kate's case, the fraud would be far less perpetuated on women of all ages everywhere.

A while back, I teamed up with a well-known trainer only to discover later that she has been bulimic for more than a decade. I then gave the job to one of America's top trainers who helped shape up some of the best bodies in Hollywood, but again, I discovered that his secret weapon was cocaine. Don't be fooled. There is no shortcut, no quick fix, no "secret" if you desire a fit and healthy body—one that will serve you well for the rest of your life.

Meanwhile, the men, women and children of America are heavier than ever. Grade school children have coronary artery disease. Our overweight and sedentary population is affecting the nation's ability to thrive as so many fall prey to physical and mental illness resulting in decreased levels of functioning.

This was so plainly evident during the Hurricane Katrina disaster. With non-stop round-the-clock coverage of the devastation, I, like many others, noticed another horror: so many people in New Orleans were overweight and obese. In fact, I heard CNN report that certain officials were concerned about people not getting their insulin medication because Louisiana has the highest rate of diabetics. Hypertension is on top of the list too. The Red Cross and shelter volunteers even made public appeals for plus-size clothing. Clearly, this is not a genetic issue but a lifestyle issue. Many may blame it on economics, but low-income lifestyles and obesity have not been linked throughout history, and such is generally not the case in other parts of the world. Evidently, it is a lack of nutritional knowledge and an indulgent and irresponsible health/information/food industry establishment that has permitted entire populations to go out of control when it comes to their weight and health issues.

In an effort to manage our weight, many of us go on diets, following fads rather than sound nutritional reality. Dieting has become a national obsession. Approximately 40% of women and 15% of men are currently on one diet or another. Even more significantly, dieting is like a rite of passage for women, with an astonishing 95% of the female population having dieted at some time in their lives. We diet in the belief that just about any diet will improve our appearance and health.

Irrefutably, dieting has a significant impact on our health, so much so that the bottom line is that our health is at stake. We know that obesity is dangerous, but the substantial risk factors imposed by the act of dieting itself threatens our good health and the health of the nation.

The national health policy regarding obesity set by the nine-member National Task Force on the Prevention and Treatment of Obesity, focused on reducing the incidence of obesity in this country by the 21st century, as noted in the document *Healthy People 2000.* This official view held by most medical professionals, including that of the Surgeon General, contends that weighing more than the ideal is unhealthy and also costly to the nation. This is a correct assumption in my view. This document focuses on the dangers of obesity, the importance of being thin, and promotes the official view that overweight people should lose weight. Yet, this document does not recognize the harm that so many fad diets may impose on many of these people.

Further, this policy does not look at the substantial increase in the prevalence of eating disorders. What is interesting about the official view is that it has been promoted by the prestigious members of the federal task force, all respected authorities on the treatment of obesity. However, a vast majority of them have financial ties with two or more commercial weight-loss firms—*each*. This tells me that the official U.S. policy regarding dieting is a bit suspect. It is a policy that primarily focuses on obesity and minimizes the risks of poor dieting choices, nutritional information, malnutrition, dysfunctional eating, and eating disorders.

> We have an
>
> abundance of
>
> food, but
>
> it is of such
>
> poor nutritional
>
> quality and
>
> so far removed
>
> from its natural
>
> state, that we
>
> are literally
>
> starving our
>
> bodies
>
> to death.

Some women feel compelled to attain the standard of beauty put forth by society. That standard idealizes thinness, thinness almost to the point of emaciation if we are to believe the messages from magazines, television, and the movies. But we are also told that in order to be healthy and to live longer, we must be at our ideal weight. Sounds good—everyone wants to be attractive and healthy. What's wrong with that? Nothing at all *if you give your body the fuel it requires.*

However, what is happening is that we are sacrificing our health in order to meet the difficult standard promoted by the diet/beauty/medical industry. An industry that garners some $50 billion annually by capitalizing on your yearning to lose weight.

The fact that we as a nation are getting fatter should come as no surprise to anyone. We are lambasted by that proclamation by articles in newspapers and magazines. Additionally, prescriptive advice aimed at us by physician-authors who for most part have *not* studied nutrition in medical school, but who do have a diet-related private practice and/or commercial products to sell you, reinforces that proclamation. We are told that we steadily grow fatter and fatter every decade. Yet surprisingly, what we are *not* told is that the increase was relatively flat from 1960 to 1980. But from 1980 to 1991, at the height of the diet and fitness craze, Americans' weight increased by eight- percent. Furthermore, that trend continues into the new millennium. In the era of low fat, no fat, sugar-free, and low carbohydrates, we are heavier and fatter than we were in Eisenhower's day.

Dieting and poor food choices are risky. Dieting causes so many problems. It can cause depression, a self-absorbed preoccupation with one's body, and food obsessions, just to name a few. It can also lead to numerous medical complications such as cardiac disorders and arrhythmia, anemia, and loss of lean body mass. Yet, the diet industry and the medical establishment would have you believe that weight loss achieved through *dieting* is necessary to reduce the risk of premature death caused primarily by cardiovascular disease. So few seem to be making the **diet** connection.

To attain optimal health is to realize that *diets don't work*. Diets cause more health problems than they solve. Something is terribly amiss. We have conquered many battles and wars during our evolutionary journey to the new millennium, but the most challenging of all may be the one that no one can escape in this modern time—*your personal body transformation*.

We live in an era of *affluent malnutrition* where 1.1 billion of the world population is obese. One out of every four *children* in America falls into this category. The rest are merely overweight with *less than five percent* of the population at a healthy weight. We have an abundance of *food*, but it is of such poor nutritional quality and so far removed from its natural state, that we are literally starving our bodies to death—whether with misguided dieting or an over-consumption of very poor food choices.

Thus, optimum health, high energy, vitality, stamina, and our passion for life are directly related to how adequately we nourish our bodies and our brains. When Hippocrates said, "Thy food will be thy remedy," he did not mean: irradiated chicken that receives an equivalent of 100,000,000 chest x-rays in radiation, bio-engineered tomatoes that carry a gene from salmon to prevent over-ripening, chemical fat substitutes that induce diarrhea, or, drinks like caffeine loaded colas and coffee, and alcohol that we consume in far excess of water—the #1 substance the brain and body needs for survival, refined sugar that damages your insulin function, or artificial sweeteners. Since your digestive system cannot metabolize artificial ingredients, it stores the unnatural substances in the fat tissues. It is generally safe there until your body utilizes its fat-stores and the chemicals are slowly released into your circulatory system, possibly causing adverse effects. It has been stated in the health community that fasting in this modern age can be dangerous because the toxins released from the fat tissue for energy during the fast, is circulated by the blood and lymphatic system throughout the body, thus weakening or poisoning the body in the process. It is best to steer clear of any artificial ingredients found in foods.

These unnatural *foods* diminish energy, put on fat, decrease your stress- capability, add cellulite, deteriorate digestion and other proper bodily functions, store toxins in your body, weaken your biological terrain and immune function, and result in a listless life, disease, premature aging and an early death. What a price to pay for your *diet*!

Fortunately, in its infinite wisdom, the body has been designed to constantly regenerate and rebuild itself. Every living cell continuously breaks down and in a normal environment, it is rebuilt. But when you consume unnatural and adulterated food—

like hormone and antibiotic-loaded meats and dairy, for example—this natural rebuilding is disrupted. As a result, cells weaken and die. When enough cells weaken and die, the body dies.

- *Every three months, you get a completely new bloodstream.*
- *Every eleven months, each cell in your body renews itself.*
- *Every two years, you get an entirely new bone structure.*

Therefore, the renewal process is taking place. Since your blood, cells and bones are constantly regenerating, *what is aging your body?*

Our ancestors primarily ate vegetables, nuts, seeds, grains, fruit, and the meat they hunted. Much of their diet was raw food. Today, scientists claim that we can live to be 150 years old given the right food selection, exercise and a safe environment. They claim that we need to return to this more natural way of eating in order to ward off disease and prevent premature aging. It is believed that premature aging and death is brought on when our body becomes so *saturated with toxic poison* that it can no longer function properly. Thus, if you *eliminate* the poison, you can control the quality and duration of your life.

In addition to large amounts of toxins found in our food, we as a nation that consume far *too much* food. Those who habitually overeat are experiencing the ultimate process of premature aging: *slow death*.

An average sedentary person simply cannot burn off the amount of calories she/he consumes. As a result, we go through life feeling tired and sick day in and day out. We are continually being medicated for headaches, indigestion, aches and pains, insomnia, allergies, blood sugar imbalances, blood pressure imbalances—the list goes on and on.

Yet, we feel the need to continue overeating in order to *maintain our strength* while our actions have the opposite effect and we burden our entire system.

When excess calories are not burned up and the process of elimination is not complete, *we become toxic.* Our body's temperature is 98.6 degrees Fahrenheit. Food that remains in the gastrointestinal tract causes toxic poisons to accumulate and autointoxication and putrefaction to set in. The toxins are then circulated throughout the body by the bloodstream, *poisoning us in the process.*

We are not left unaware of this process. From bad breath to poor skin to headaches to indigestion to aches and pains—these are just a few of the symptoms that many of us experience at one time or another. Depression, moodiness, sleep disturbances, irritability and the inability to control common stress, are all too familiar.

When enervation cripples the eliminative functions, this affects not only the bowels, but your liver, kidneys, skin, and lungs. Collectively, they make for a tired, sick, lifeless individual.

The body has been known to take years and years of abuse. But left to continuous deteriorating habits, in time, *restitution*

Today, scientists claim that we can live to be 150 years old given the right food selection, exercise, and a safe environment.

14

makes its claim. In order for vital force—the energy of youth—to be restored, we need to make smarter dietary selections.

Edmund Bordeaux Szchely carried out extensive research on the Dead Sea Scrolls and found that the Essenes, compilers of the Scrolls in the last centuries of the pre-Christian era, divided foods into categories based on what they perceived as their inherent energies.

Biogenic (from the ancient Greek meaning "life-generating") foods are those that can be planted to produce more foods—for example seeds, whole grains, nuts, and pulses (crops harvested solely for their dry grain).

Bioactive foods, they said, provide nourishment to the human body and sustain it, but they cannot generate new life—fruits and vegetables.

Biostatic foods are neither life-generating nor life-sustaining and they slow down life processes in the body—cooked foods and those that are not fresh.

Finally, *biocidic* ("life-destroying") foods are actually harmful to the body. In the modern diet, these would include foods containing additives and preservatives and those that have been refined and otherwise far removed from nature. In other words, pretty much what you would find in a general grocery store today.

Other cultures went even further than the Essene community and used food specifically as medicine. It was the basis of medicine in ancient Egypt, Babylonia, Greece and China, and in Europe during the Middle Ages. It has been only within the last 100 years—and particularly the last 50—that the industrial societies of the world have become dependent on artificially manufactured drugs to cure illness. Today, prescription drugs are one of the top leading causes of death. Certain drugs worked wonderfully against infections that caused many deaths in the past. Now, those drugs have been signally unsuccessful against the same infections.

I repeat, we suffer from *affluent malnutrition*. We have an abundance of food available to us, but so little of it is *life-promoting*. As a result, many experts claim that for some people, stopping the eating of junk food can equate to getting off alcohol or other abused substances. The withdrawal symptoms can be rough and a series of healing crises usually occur as the body detoxifies.

For this reason, many people give up early in the process, thus never allowing themselves the opportunity to transform their bodies and reach optimal health and youthful energy. We all know of individuals who boast about their deplorable eating habits and say they still feel terrific! I challenged such a person. Anna is an attractive, energetic and successful 36-year-old attorney who continuously mocked and ridiculed my choices about what I would and would not eat. "I'm perfectly happy with Big Macs, French fries, Coke, and coffee," she would remind me enthusiastically at every opportunity. "I like a bowl of ice cream while unwinding in front of the television before going to bed," she would add. So I asked her to go without her favorite foods for just one week and see what would happen. "No problem!" She readily agreed in her usual cheerful and carefree manner.

She didn't last a week, however. She lasted *two* days! Headaches, leg cramps, drowsiness, and irritability forced her back on her junk food diet.

Eliminating poisons, improving your digestion, and introducing vital nutrients to your blood, cells, and bones can be a bumpy experience during transition. Side effects of detoxification can include headaches, muscle aches, indigestion, nausea, temperature imbalance, depression, and irritability, among other symptoms, depending on how toxic you are. But these symptoms usually subside from several days to several months, depending on your level of toxicity and biological individuality.

In time, as you eliminate processed and artificial foods from your diet and replace them with the fresh and wholesome variety, you will notice a visible change in your skin, muscle tone, energy level and general mood. You will feel rejuvenated and will notice a sunnier disposition as well as increased mental clarity. Some people mark the change as downright miraculous. You begin by avoiding the foods that are robbing you of optimal health and then you detoxify your system, which takes away the aches, pains and mood swings as it brings on restored energy and optimism. For most of us, it is worth the effort to own a clean, painless, tireless and ageless body. After all—*youthfulness is internal purity.*

CHAPTER 2
ATTITUDE TRANSFORMATION

Transforming your body often means transforming your life. Think about it: at what point do you begin to live your life backwards? I think this happens when poor dietary choices become the centerpiece of your life. Food is designed to enhance life. It is an important part of life. When you start to put your food preferences before your health and appearance, before the quality of living, you lose out on life.

We don't have a problem with deciding to go on a diet. As you already know, we have become a nation of professional dieters. More than two-thirds of Americans are overweight, some 40% are obese; however, more than half of them are making absolutely no effort to lose weight. And with good reason: diets don't work. The National Institutes of Health (NIH) reports that 95% of dieters regain all of their lost weight within 12 to 36 months after dieting. Instead, what's really at issue here is a problem with *food control.*

Many of us understand this all too well. Eating is an emotional issue for most people. As one friend stated, "If someone hurts me, I have a tendency to hurt myself by overeating *comfort* foods."

So many of us were rewarded with food throughout life, especially with sweets when we were young. It is no wonder that we turn to "comfort foods" now when we want to feel better. Some of us never fully realize to what extent emotional eating runs our lives.

Problems with food control lead to a host of ailments which needlessly forces us to face premature aging, and not just weight gain. The NIH claims that even five to ten pounds more than the optimal weight could cause health problems. NIH goes on to explain that the link between obesity and premature death has actually been underestimated. It seems that the only way people can be successful at losing weight and enjoying robust health is to change their attitudes and beliefs.

When your body and mind work together, you become aware of the difference between your body's true nutritional needs and emotional or stress-induced false alarms. In fact, proponents of mind and body therapies claim that the body has an *inner intelligence* to keep it in perfect health. This intelligence also monitors how, when and what you should eat— to be slim, to be healthy, to be energized, to live a long life. The key is to pay attention to your inner intelligence.

Even five to ten pounds more than the optimal weight could cause health problems.

"This inner intelligence even governs how food is consumed and converted to energy," said the famed health guru, Dr. Deepak Chopra. "When that intelligence is ignored, the body's mechanics are thrown off balance."

But why is there so much obesity in the United States and not the rest of the world? Why is there a 30 percent increase in obesity among children in the United States in the past decade? Are we simply more out of touch with this inner intelligence?

For one, our consumption of snacks has a direct correlation to the rate of obesity. This is *subconscious eating*. In the United States, more than in any other country, we have 24-hour food stores and restaurants. Convenience and availability has a lot to do with consumption. A lot of our eating is out of habit and as a response to external cues. It has nothing to do with being hungry. That's why those people who think the problem of being overweight will be found in appetite control just don't get it! Most people who are overweight are not eating because they are hungry; they are eating what they like for reasons such as *food preference*.

Once you become aware of intuitive eating and hunger, dietary practices will not be a complicated issue. When we recognize that *food is nothing more than fuel*, this will distance us from emotional urges to eat. Just ask yourself how many times you ate mindlessly while reading, at the theater or sporting event, or watching television. Did you want the crunch, the smoothness, the chewiness, the saltiness, the sweetness? Did it have anything to do with hunger or nutritional need? Most likely, it did not. It is important to note that people who practice conscious eating notice that they are eating from one-third to one-half less than they used to, and feel more satisfied.

In order to understand our food control problem, we have to understand the origins of our eating philosophy. American society was founded by people who came here not only seeking political freedom, but freedom from hunger. They brought with them a value system that glorified food and they taught us that it is a sin to waste and to throw food away. From their origins, as a society where there was food depravation, it would be a sin to throw food away because that may be a difference between life and death.

But in our society, we have an abundance of food that has been disastrously combined with the fact that we are the children of these ancestors and still maintain their value system. If you can't eat it, it's deprivation. You can't throw it out; it's a waste. But in reality, we are throwing out our bodies, our health, and our appearance. The sin now is to consume the excess and to throw out our health and the hopes of a long and productive future.

What helps us about the Transformation food program is that it is *not a diet but a new value system.* The diet imposes a structure on eating so you're not out of control. If you look at all the diets, they basically come down to the same

> People often eat when they are lonely, frustrated, sad, anxious or angry, choosing food in response to emotional rather than physical needs.

foods. Diets set a structure for eating that's out of control and that's why diets work—but they don't last. People do not seek weight control because they are happy people. They seek it because they're unhappy. As soon as the weight starts to go down, unless they come to understand the role of their attitudes and their feelings about food, and unless they realize what so many people in our society don't want to comprehend—that *you lose the weight but you don't lose the problem*. Unless they can understand these dynamics, all of their weight loss efforts are only temporary. Even America's most famous dieter agrees that you must resolve any underlying emotional baggage first. Oprah Winfrey said, "Fear, specifically of not being liked and the fear of saying no," prevented her from making needed changes in her lifestyle.

So, how do we go about changing these value systems? First of all, we have to recognize that it's not just a problem with nutritional information that we have. Most of us in middle class and upper middle class society, who have weight problems, already know what to eat and what not to eat. You know when you eat the wrong food, so it's not a problem with nutritional information. We are an educated society. We are not our great-grandparents who didn't know that chocolate is high in fat; who didn't know that certain foods are high in cho-lesterol. We have nutritional information but it's a matter of making it a lifestyle. To achieve that goal you have to recog-nize the impact: this is a food-oriented society. Even the lan-guage of love is food oriented—honey, sweetie, cookie.

We have become a *foodie culture*. It's a culture that glori-fies food. We are very food centered and we believe that as a part of this foodie orientation, we should be able to have it all. If we can't have a certain food because of health reasons or because of a history of abusing it, then we feel deprived!

We have to work on our own value system and we have to grow up in the area of food and realize that most of us, as we age, cannot have it all and still be slim, fit and healthy. This is not a nutritional and weight control principle, it is a principle of reality. *If you want a scenario for unhappiness, approach life with the value system that you can have it all.*

Even in our relationships with the people that we love— family, friends, employees—we cannot have it all. Most of us have accepted this, albeit not happily, in all other areas of living. It's only in the area of food that we want to have it all and still expect to be thin and healthy and to age beautifully. We cannot change the principles of reality that apply to 95% of us. Five percent of the population has it as their birthright to eat whatever they want while seemingly getting away with it. But for the rest of us, with the slowing down of metabolic efficacy as we get older, we cannot have it all. *Our attitudes and our feelings are as important as our nutritional knowledge.*

Furthermore, we also have to take a closer look at *personality*. To think that our eating exists in a vacuum when everything else in our life is accepted by our personality is an injustice. To think that personality does not exude influence on eating behavior is to be profoundly naive.

It seems that we have all other parts of our life under control but not food: *what makes a success makes an excess.* The critical thing to understand both in terms of longevity and biological function is that it's excessiveness that ruins the fun of life and the length of life. If we want to age well, we have to watch for excessiveness in terms of eating.

People who could be happy with a little, could never be very successful. The same qualities that propel a person to achieve on that high level also propels them to excessive behavior and even addictive and destructive behavior. It seems that is where we get the expression that genius contains the seed of its own destruction. The very qualities that enable a person to possess such intensity in one part of their life can also result in excessive eating, drug or alcohol abuse. With that kind of intensity, you will destroy yourself. Thus, we may conclude that *the successful personality is often more prone to excessive behavior.*

Hence, the reason so many people have trouble with weight issues and with managing their weight is that they simply don't manage and plan their eating as they manage and plan other parts of their life. Consequently, eating becomes an unplanned, undisciplined, haphazard occurrence. A number of hours pass and without a planned meal, a person will grab whatever is around. When we drive our car, we plan on stopping for gas. The human body is also a machine and unless you understand that you have to stop every few hours for refueling, your eating becomes more and more compulsive and less and less controlled. So needless to say, you cannot eat properly without planning: buying the right foods and having them available.

Think of thin as we get older as a learned skill. When we were young, for many of us it was our birthright, but as we get older, we come back to the evolutionary theory of Darwin: *those who can adapt endure; those who cannot adapt parish.* In a very real sense, eating to transform your body is based on that philosophy. As we age, our body is losing metabolic efficacy and the only way we can get around it is through certain types of foods.

In addition, the human personality also tends to want bountiful *quantity*. Human beings do not like to be given small servings of food. We are a hunter-gatherer people and we tend to value quantity. That is why if you look at the biggest range in the restaurant food industry, it's those restaurants that serve family style. So, we have to look at our psychology *and* biology. If you want quantity, you can still have quantity if you understand food quality and food control in respect to life preservation. It is much easier to control your weight that way than to live your life backwards.

This is no simple task in today's overabundant commercial society. But if you look at the fittest people, they are always a small number among us. *The norm does not usually do too well in terms of revolution.* After all, to worry about being normal is the preoccupation of the insecure. What is normal for us is what works for our bodies. If you look at the field of nutrition, you will notice that it has changed often. Therefore, what we have to go on is this guideline: your body is a text book for *you*.

The goal that I have for you with this book, is that *you achieve your own personal best*. The very best you can do given

Any food that you cannot control is controlling you.

your genetic endowment, your personal life circumstances and your socioeconomic group. Given the circumstances of your life, the goal is to strive for your personal best.

As we become more aware of our full potential to achieve body transformation, we must acknowledge our own *eating print*, a signature eating pattern. This usually leads to serious weight and health problems when neglected. Putting aside the food quality issue for the moment, let's deal with those of us who don't appear to understand why we have problems with food control—perhaps the ultimate cause of premature aging. After all, we didn't become overweight, under-energized and unmotivated because we ate far too many fresh vegetables and fish. If you're anything like me, you have probably gained weight on high sugar, high fat, high starch treats that culture and society tell us are good; the foods that cause more illness and death in our society than any virus.

The first and foremost strategy of weight loss can be summarized in these words: *learn from your history!*

Every person who lost weight and gained it back did so with the very same types of food, at the very same times of day, week, month, and year that had caused them to gain weight in the first place. *Whenever you go back to your old pattern, the weight, and the problems associated with it, come back.*

No matter what your age, ethnic background, religion or nationality, your weight problem is the result of a combination of biological, psychological behavior and emotional elements that work together to determine your food choices. If you want to change your weight, you need to recognize and change your *eating pattern*.

You may diet, you may fast, but ultimately you will return to the pattern of your eating print—unless you learn to permanently avoid and control these triggers.

There is a probability attached to each food you eat. Some of us have a high probability that we will lose control, some of us a low one. A particular food may trigger your appetite to such a degree that even when you try to control the amount you eat, you fail. Or it may be a food that you always turn to in times of stress. Or it may even be a type of food (like finger foods) that, once you start, you feel compelled to keep eating, regardless of whether you are hungry or even like it!

Been there done that? I certainly have—more times than I care to admit. You undoubtedly already know the foods you like and are inclined to overindulge in. You may even recognize some of the behaviors and situations that prompt you to overeat. What I recommend that you need to do is to put it all together to see the probabilities of an overall *pattern* to your behavior. Your *eating print* is the mirror in which you can see your eating history.

Prevention is the cure and your eating print is the prescription. It will shape every aspect of your weight loss and diet plan to choosing a specific food.

A sure way for prevention to work is to accurately identify your *trigger foods*. Trigger foods are the ones that you can't have just one of—once you've started, you won't stop until the supply runs out. Sound familiar? These are the foods that prompt *chain eating*.

Perhaps you think that ALL foods are your trigger foods! These people believe that when they start eating, they are unable to stop—no matter what the food. But most people with food control problems are actually susceptible to a relatively small number of very specific foods, usually pretty unhealthy ones.

Most people can easily identify their trigger foods. But if you aren't sure of yours, start by making a list of all of your favorite foods. Do you notice a pattern? Do any of the foods belong to a specific food category? What have these foods done for you? All they have done, I'm willing to bet the ranch, is add pounds to your weight, take years off your life, and erode your sense of self-worth and self-esteem. *Any food that you cannot control is controlling you.* You must ask yourself: what is the true cost of eating this food for my weight, my health and my life?

Some people call this phenomenon *food addiction* because it is so similar to other addictive processes. Like drugs, trigger foods have a destructive effect on your behavior, causing you to lose control despite your determination not to.

Thin is not free! There is a price, and it may be the elimination of some of your trigger foods from your diet. In addition to identifying our trigger foods, I want you to understand The Great Lie. Perhaps the greatest threat to maintaining control over trigger foods is the phrase that I like to call, The Great Lie of Dieting: "I'll have just a little!"

No, you don't have to be unreasonably hard on yourself. Logically, an intelligent, motivated person should be able to taste any old problem food and then stop at a little. But reality and logic are rarely in agreement. You can't control a trigger food with logic alone. Taste buds have a memory and a power all of their own!

So beware of even your best intentions. Like the road to hell, the road to fat is paved with good intentions. Therefore, it appears that we have no choice but to steer clear of The Great Lie. Tell yourself: "If I don't take the first little taste, I don't begin. Thus, I don't have a problem."

In the area of trigger foods there can be no equivocation. If a specific food or type of food threatens the quality of your life, don't go there. That food has to be sent packing. If you are absolutely unable to eat it in moderation at any time in your life, then you should not eat it at all. After all, no one who lost and then regained weight ever said, "I think I'll start over-eating again so I can get fat." If such were the case, I could write the sequel, "Now That You're Thin, Begin Again!" If 95% of dieters have been proven wrong, do you really think you will be **The One** to beat the odds?

Control is just like a muscle—the more you exercise it by saying, "No, thank you," the stronger you become and the easier it becomes to say, "No, thank you," in the future.

When trigger foods and The Big Lie are under control, I must warn you against *trigger behavior*. This is the habitual and often virtually unconscious behavioral pattern that leads to the repeated abuse of

Remind yourself of what food did and did not do for you in the past: It did make you fat and it did not make you happy.

the trigger foods that make you fat. Trigger behaviors can be hard to pin down, since so many of them are subconscious. The calories are popped into your mouth by the thousands and never register in your mind, although they certainly do register on your backside!

Those with trigger behavior are labeled as a Picker, Prowler, Finisher, or Hoarder. Most dieters are Pickers: people who love finger foods of any kind and who can go through thousands of calories within minutes. I'm a reformed Picker myself. Finger foods are the Picker's worst enemy, which is why I say that more people have gained weight with their fingers than with their mouths.

If you are a Picker, I advise that the essence of weight control is finger control. More people have gained weight from what they eat before, after and in-between meals, than from what they consume at the meal itself.

And then, we must consider *trigger emotions*. Sometimes eating or feeling hungry is not about food. *People often eat when they are lonely, frustrated, sad, anxious, or angry, choosing food in response to emotional rather than physical needs.*

Food is clearly more comforting to some people than it is to others. Instead of coping with painful or difficult emotions, they use food as a panacea. When the going gets tough, they stuff. Those who have difficulty with trigger emotions have developed a one-word response to any and all problems: EAT!

If you turn to food for solace, you are confusing pleasure with long-term happiness. These eating episodes are "destructive pleasures." After all, *whenever you mistake immediate gratification for happiness, you are risking the length and quality of your life for a few seconds or minutes of pleasure.*

As long as your eating is tied to your emotions, you will never achieve a stable weight. Your weight will change as often as your emotions do. And any diet—no matter how sound—will be as futile as trying to build a castle in the sand. It will be swept away with the next wave of emotion.

You deserve better than that and you can have it. Just as you can become more physically fit through exercise and healthy living, you can become more psychologically fit. You can learn the difference between coping and consumption, between instant gratification and happiness. You can learn to manage your weight by learning to manage your life—without turning to food. After all, if you control an empire but feel out of control with your own body, how can you truly enjoy your success?

Consider the following questions:

- *What kind of "reward" makes you miserable five minutes later?*
- *What kind of "treat" makes you throw out the clothes you love?*
- *What kind of "cure" ruins your looks, your health, and your self-esteem?*

You can use the knowledge of your *eating print* to become a good self-therapist, to spot the trouble situations and behaviors before they occur and take steps to protect yourself. And by understanding your eating print you can better *remind yourself of what food did and did not do for you in the past: It did make you fat and it did not make you happy.*

Therefore, you must consistently ask yourself: What food or foods always seem to prompt you to uncontrolled eating? In what situations? In what moods? Does your favorite food serve as a trigger only when you actually have it in the house?

Do you lose control of it only when you are angry or stressed? Use your eating print to shed light on the overall pattern of your eating history. More than likely, you will see that you are not out of control with "food" in general, but only with a few "select foods," in very specific situations.

Your eating print is more than a window onto your past, it is also a crystal ball to your future. If your eating print shows that you consistently abused a food in the past, you can know with certainty that you will abuse it in the future.

CHAPTER 3
MIND TRANSFORMATION

Nothing stands still. It never did and it never will. While virtually all physical matter appears motionless to the naked human eye, in reality, there is no solid physical matter whatsoever. The hardest piece of steel is just a well orchestrated mass of revolving particles. As we know, the unseen atom is nature's building block from which becomes a tree, a stone, my cat, and Gucci shoes. ALL matter is in a consistent state of vibration—it literally moves non-stop. The molecule consists of fast moving particles we call atoms, and atoms are made up of fast moving particles named electrons.

Within every single particle of matter lies an unseen force which makes the atoms circle around each other at an unimaginable speed. A single rate of vibration produces sound. Our ears can detect only the sound that comes from 20 to 20,000 cycles per second. As the cycles increase, they are manifested as heat. Go farther up the scale, vibrations or cycles register in the form of light. This includes the invisible ultraviolet rays and energy with a wavelength of an even higher order, also cannot be seen although the heat sure can be felt!

Progressing up the scale, the vibrations continue to create the power, many advanced thinking individuals believe, with

which people *think*. Whether you sub-
scribe to the Biblical teaching or scientific
discovery, *thoughts are energy*. Hence, if we
are to take a lesson from chemistry in this
instance, we can conclude that the only difference among thoughts, sound, heat or
light is the number of vibrations per second. It also means that thought travels,
affects, and has consequences.

Perhaps Alexander Graham Bell
posed the question best. "If the thought
waves are similar to the wireless waves,
they must pass from the brain and flow
endlessly around the world and the uni-
verse. The body and the skull and other
solid obstacles would form no obstruction
to their passage, as they pass through the
ether that surrounds the molecules of
every substance, no matter how solid or
dense. Thus, you ask if there would not be
constant interference and confusion if
other people's thoughts were flowing
through our brains and setting up thoughts
in them that did not originate with ourselves?" Ah, there lies the secret!

Bell posed questions that may
already be a reality while science catches
up. Hence, we have to ask ourselves, to
what extent are our thoughts affecting our
physical and mental well being? To what
extent are we responsible for our well-

Optimists have fewer incidents of stress-related illnesses. When they do succumb to sickness, they recover much faster.

being when we expose ourselves to the ideas, images and interactions that we engage in every day? How is our rightful thinking, or alternatively as minister and popular author, Joyce Meyer would say, "stinkin' thinkin'," determining the precise course of our lives? How do you know that the thoughts of others are not interfering with yours now?

Bell stated that scientific discoveries will soon bring us to a point when we will be able to read one another's thoughts and when thoughts will be conveyed directly from brain to brain without intervention of speech, writing, or any of the present known methods of communication.

"The hypothesis that mind can communicate directly with mind rests on the theory that thought or vital force is a form of electrical disturbance, that it can be taken up by induction and transmitted to a distance either through a wire or simply through the all-pervading ether, as in the case of wireless telegraph waves," Bell stated.

It is possible to cite many reasons why thought and vital force may be regarded as of the same nature as electricity. As Bell explained, the electric current is held to be a wave motion of ether, the hypothetical substance that fills all space and pervades all substances. It is believed there must be ether because without it the electric current could not pass through a vacuum, or sunlight through space. It is reasonable to believe that the only wave motion of a similar character can produce the phenomena of thought and vital force. We may assume that the brain cells act as a battery and that the current produced flows along the nerves.

Thus, we may conclude that every single mind is a broadcasting *and* receiving station! If we comprehended this and applied it even fractionally to our daily lives, how differently would we think and feel? Thomas Paine stated it very well, "Any person who made observations of the state of progress of the human mind by observing his own, cannot but have observed that there are two distinct classes of thoughts: those that we produce ourselves by reflection and act of thinking, and those that bolt into the mind of their own accord. Every person of learning is finally his own teacher...."

Considering what science knows today and what may be eventually proven by Bell's theory, can one reasonably ask if there is a link between your thoughts and your health? Current research certainly suggests so. In plain and direct language, positive thinking people simply have a better attitude, better health and live longer. It has been determined that how we cope with stress depends on our attitude. On the flip side, attitude also affects the way stress manages us. Think of it as a criminal who knows how to pick his prey. Those who are more vulnerable are more likely to be victims.

Rightful thinking optimists are better able to handle stressful situations. Optimists have less incidents of developing a stress-related illness. When they do succumb to sickness, they recover much faster.

On the other hand, those engaged in constant negative thinking tend to deny their problems, they remove themselves from having to deal with stressful issues, they dwell on stressful feelings, and perhaps most detrimentally, they permit the stressful situation to interfere with the accomplishment of a goal. Pessimists are generally more ill than the optimists among us. They even use defeatist language to express themselves like, "I can't," which states powerlessness, while "I won't" expresses a choice.

Stress is the major culprit of the new millennium. Simply defined, stress is the body's response to any demand made upon it. Stress used to be a matter of survival. An increased pulse, fast and shallow breathing, a heightened state of alertness was what kept our ancestors away from danger and ready to fight or flee.

Today, stress comes in a multitude of fronts and guises—good and bad. Marriage is a stressful situation, as is a financial crisis or a death in the family. But then there is the real killer, the chronic low-grade stress that comes from not being able or willing to properly manage life as we're living it. The symptoms are all too evident: depression, sadness, anxiety, an unreasonable fear, tension, nervousness, anger, hostility, panic, a feeling of loosing control or even aloofness, sarcasm, and rudeness towards others. As the commercial states, social anxiety disorders!

Not all stress is bad, however. It sure can motivate some of us to do better, work smarter, and challenge ourselves to new heights. This can result in a better life. Researchers have concluded that it's not necessarily the stressful event that affects us, but how we respond to that event. For instance, what one person perceives as very stressful can challenge him to victory while it can totally cripple another person.

The link between personality and health is all too real. The latest studies show that optimism and a sunny disposition goes a good way to contributing to not just a healthier life but a long life as well. There is a body of evidence that well-adjusted, socially stable, well-integrated and content people have a lower risk of disease and premature death than loners and the chronically discontented and pessimistic. Much of the research states that optimism is associated with increased longevity. In a 23-year study of residents in one small Ohio town by researchers from Yale and Miami Universities, those over the age of 50 who viewed aging as a positive experience lived an average of 7.5 years longer than those who dreaded getting old. In fact, people did better with optimism than with life-prolonging medications in some instances, like lowering elevated blood cholesterol.

Mayo Clinic researchers tracked 447 people whose personal traits had been studied 30 years earlier. Those classified as optimists had half the risk of premature death compared to those classified as pessimistic or mixed. The optimists had fewer problems as they aged, fewer limitations, less pain, and more energy.

The University of Texas found that people with an upbeat view of life where less likely than pessimists to show signs of frailty. They speculate that positive emotions may directly affect health by altering the chemical balance of the body.

"Is the Glass Half Empty or Half Full?" was a study conducted by Harvard researcher Dr. Laura Kubzansky, who found that optimism, as determined by the way people justify the events in their lives, was protective against heart disease. But when they did succumb to heart disease, other studies show that optimists recover faster after coronary bypass surgery than the negative thinkers. In fact, many

> The mental health community issued a report stating that in less than a decade, more than 50% of the American population will be diagnosed with one type of mental illness or another.

researchers have come to the conclusion that negative emotions and chronic pessimism should be regarded as a risk factor for heart disease.

Personality can alter health and life expectancy in so many ways. Chronic frustration and anger may lead to smoking, drinking, bad eating habits or drug abuse. An optimistic person is more likely to be motivated to change self-destructive habits or better yet, not engage in them in the first place. An optimistic individual is also more likely to seek medical attention and seek to prevent a physical or mental breakdown of any kind while a negative person will avoid facing potentially troublesome symptoms. Furthermore, it is well documented that optimism has a positive impact on the immune system. Thus, you can literally "think" yourself well or ill—completely or in degrees—given the right or wrong mindset.

That said, the personality trait most associated with longevity is "conscientiousness," according to researchers at the University of California at Riverside. Conscientiousness is defined as self-discipline, dependability, prudence, care, and the will to achieve. These traits are certainly more important over the course of a lifetime, but it is never too late to apply them. While thinking carefully before you act is not the same thing as optimism, conscientiousness is a sound and realistic underpinning for optimism.

How happy are you? Are you in need of a mind transformation? If you watch the popular reality television shows these days, you know that anything is possible with the right makeover. A happiness makeover, however, may be the most extreme of all because unless you're naturally optimistic, or you are a Disney Princess, it's a constant learning and applying process.

Transforming what you can't see on the inside is the ultimate makeover indeed.

The National Institute on Aging recently funded a project with the objective of creating a "National Well-Being Account." This was designed to help supplement the GNP, the great statistical machine that counts goods and services. The researchers concluded that big measurements of health and wealth don't tell the whole story about how happy people are in America. They reported that we may be struggling with the "hedonic treadmill." It's a phenomenon observed in the developed world and it basically means that the more you have, the more you want, and that even a large increase in income does not usually increase life satisfaction.

Unfortunately, in this modern age where we usually have an abundance of information and options if a lack of self-governance, instead of going to the root of the problem, many people needlessly turn to antidepressants as they are so readily available and often pushed by their physicians. The promise is often greater than the reality as so many people are not mentally ill as they are ill-equipped to handle life's many stressful situations. While some are genuinely in need of psychiatric medications, most are not. Even the most

> With every thought you think and every bite you put into your mouth, you are either generating life or pursuing death.

liberal among us has to raise an eyebrow when the mental health community issues a report stating that in less than a decade, more than 50 percent of the American population will be diagnosed with one type of mental illness or another. That can only be great news if you're a pharmaceutical company share holder!

There are many ways of treating depression and various anxiety disorders, and chief among them are nutrition and dietary supplements. London's Brain Bio Center has reported the use of a radical therapy—*food*. Last August, CBS News reported that "thousands of Britons suffering from depression, mental illness, and even attention deficit disorder are now, *controversially*, looking to nutritional therapy as a path to wellness."

Their "food for better mood" crusade claims that diet can be fine-tuned to influence brain chemistry. The center reports that most of their patients reduce or go off the medication after a year-long food and supplement regimen.

CBS further reported that three clinical studies in Britain, Israel, and the United States show there is something to this. Increased intake of omega-3 fatty acids found in fish (even with the mercury found in fish issue, the latest research claims that it is safe to consume up to 12 ounces per week without any adverse effects) had what researchers describe as "a substantial impact" on depression and bi-polar disorder. There has been much concern in recent times among the general public regarding the safety of fish due to its reported high mercury content. However, the latest research claims that the benefits of eating fish far outweigh any risk from trace amounts of mercury.

The Harvard Center for Risk Analysis in October 2005 conducted a study, "A Quantitative Analysis of the Risks and Benefits Associated with Changes in Fish Consumption," that was published in November by the American Journal of

Preventive Medicine. The study concludes women of childbearing age and pregnant women can eat up to 12 ounces of fish per week with no negative impact. (The risks from mercury in fish and shellfish depend on the amount of fish and shellfish eaten. Therefore pregnant women, women who might become pregnant, nursing mothers, and young children should avoid some types of fish such as shark, swordfish, King mackerel, Tilefish, and Albacore tuna. They should instead eat canned light tuna, salmon, Pollock, and catfish, which are lower in mercury.)

This study further warned that reduced fish consumption will result in serious public health consequences, including higher death rates from heart disease and stroke.

While this is news to the mainstream media, those who have sought out and practiced nutritional and natural remedies have been aware of this for ages.

But the powers that be persist. One of the most mind-boggling pieces of information that I have come across was a BBC News report from August 8, 2004 with its headline: *Prozac "found in drinking water."* The story went on to say that an Environment Agency report suggests so many people are taking the drug nowadays it is building up in rivers and groundwater! A spokesman for the Drinking Water Inspectorate said, "The Prozac found was most likely highly diluted." Huh? Is this the new fluoride?

The Sunday Observer said the environmentalists were calling for an urgent investigation into the evidence. It quotes the Liberal Democrats' environment spokesman as saying the picture emerging looked like "a case of hidden mass medication upon the unsuspecting public." He went on to say "it's alarming that there is no monitoring of levels of Prozac and other pharmacy residues in our drinking water." The BBC states that the antidepressant drug gets into the rivers and water systems via treated sewage water. They report that the exact amount of Prozac in the nation's drinking water is not known. At the same time, the Environment Agency report concluded that the Prozac in the water table could be potentially toxic and said the drug was a "potential concern."

While the officials are *potentially concerned*, when it comes to your well-being and longevity, the buck stops with you. In Britain alone, from 1991 to 2001, the number of prescriptions for antidepressants went up from nine million per year to 24 million per year. Those figures are even more staggering in the United States. This many people couldn't possibly be out of their right mind. Something is clearly amiss in the way we view our body, mind, and spirit.

We are built to perfection. Every normal human body has a high-tech chemical laboratory and a warehouse of chemicals sufficient to carry on the business of breaking up, assimilating, and properly mixing and compounding the food we eat, and distributing it to wherever it is needed by the body for optimal functioning.

Our thoughts and emotions from the energy we call the mind, play a vital part in this chemical operation of compounding and transforming food into the necessary substances to build and keep the body—which includes the brain—in good working order. All forms of anxiety will undoubtedly interfere with the digestive process. In extreme cases, this process will stop altogether—gastritis at best, death at worst. What more proof do you then require that the mind enters into the chemistry of food digestion, assimilation, and ultimate nourishment?

When the mind becomes consumed with negative thoughts, the entire nervous system can be thrown out of order. As digestion is disturbed, various diseases can begin to manifest themselves. The culprits that are most detrimental to such emotional turmoil stand the test of time—financial problems and unrequited love.

The chemistry of mind will further destruct in a negative environment. A nagging spouse, a lack of balance in one's activities, a lack of purpose or satisfaction about one's circumstances can make a person lose ambition and cause them to gradually sink into oblivion.

Back to nourishment, today almost all of us know that certain food combinations inevitably result in indigestion, pain, certain allergic reactions, and so forth. Just watch television for an hour and see how many medications are advertised for the troublesome symptoms resulting from your diet. Countless drugs for indigestion, bloating, gas, acid reflux disease, the list goes on and on. If you need to medicate yourself every time you eat, something is terribly amiss.

Good health, good mood and longevity depend, to a reasonable extent, on a food combination that is harmonious with your body's requirements not just to survive but to thrive. Harmony appears to be one of nature's basic laws without which there can be no energy or life in any form at all. The health of your body and that of your mind is literally created from the principle of harmony. The energy we call life begins to diminish and death nears closer when the organs of the body cease to work in harmony. Thus, with every thought you think and every bite you put into your mouth, you are either generating life or pursuing death. The good news is—you have options; the decision is yours.

CHAPTER 4
THE BODY TRANSFORMATION
FOOD GUIDE PYRAMID

As we begin to transform our bodies, we must transform some dietary myths that have been dictated to us as vital guidelines by "experts" and endorsed as such by our government.

I often find myself in a state of total disbelief when I encounter incredibly gifted, intelligent and accomplished individuals who are absolutely clueless about their food choices. I am dumbstruck by the contents of most people's grocery carts at any given supermarket.

Recently, I found myself behind a young mother at an Albertson's checkout counter who was desperately trying to stop her two small children from going ape in the aisles. She commented to bewildered onlookers that it's always like this. She even volunteered that she had an older child confined at home because of his uncontrollable hyperactivity and unpredictable outbursts.

I glanced at her over-flowing cart only to note enough of a junk food and chemical brew worthy of being classified as bodily weapons of mass destruction. I dared to ask if this was standard fare in her household. "Oh, they won't eat anything else!" was her defiant reply. She actually seemed to take offense that

I dared to imply anything concerning her food selections. Clearly, the lack of nutrients has affected her attitude and personality as well.

Although there is no shortage of dietary information out there, as is evident by the tens of millions of diet books that are sold annually, it is quite staggering to realize just how few people want to be bothered when it comes to changing their food choices.

The adamant that want to change and become informed health consumers are frequently bombarded with only some truths, loads of half-truths and far too many outright lies. There is no lack of misinformation in the dietary world, that is for certain.

Let's consider a major half-truth: the USDA Food Guide Pyramid, which is the government prescribed food eating recommendations in America. It is officially defined as a diagrammatic representation of human nutritional needs devised by the U.S. Department of Agriculture in 1992 and updated, albeit poorly in January 2005. It replaced the "four food groups" pie chart used since the 1950s. The USDA "Food Guide Pyramid," until very recently, featured a relatively wide base of 6-11 servings daily of grains and cereals beneath a

Only 9% of Americans eat the necessary five or more servings of fruits and vegetables a day.

layer representing 5-9 servings daily of fruits and vegetables. A third level represents 4-6 daily servings of meats and dairy products. At the peak of the Pyramid are fats and sweets, to be eaten sparingly.

On the surface, all appeared somewhat sound. However, when you began to examine this more closely and realized that it was just the same old processed sugar and chemical loaded "food," you felt quite differently.

The USDA defended its creation by explaining that the Pyramid is an outline of what to eat each day. It is not a rigid prescription but a general guide that lets you choose a healthy diet that's right for you. Granted, the Pyramid is intended for the widest possible audience and you must take your own common sense and biological individuality into consideration. Otherwise, it's sort of like everyone wearing the same size bra or dentures—small adjustment, big difference.

Neither the previous nor the current Pyramid sits well with most health authorities. The horror is that the official government Pyramid (currently called MyPyramid) is taught in schools, appears in countless media articles and broadcasts, and is plastered on cereal boxes and food labels. The Harvard School of Public Health reports that, "Technically, the information embodied in this Pyramid didn't point the way to healthy eating." Since this is what it was created to do, why not? "It's blueprint was based on shaky scientific evidence, and it barely changed over the years to reflect major advances in our understanding of the connection between diet and health," Harvard experts concluded.

Nevertheless, with much fanfare, the USDA finally put to rest the old Food Guide Pyramid and presented the public with MyPyramid. They gave us a new rainbow pyramid symbol and an "interactive food guidance system" that can only be obtained on-line. The new symbol is primarily the old Pyramid turned on its side.

The Harvard School of Public Health issued a report stating, in part, "It continues to recommend foods that aren't essential to good health, and may even be detrimental in the quantities included in MyPyramid."

Unfortunately, the USDA's My Pyramid had many architects—those both evident and below the radar. The nutritionists, staffers, and consultants were intertwined with the determined lobbyists from a smorgasbord of food industries. Federal regulations dictate that the panel that creates and writes the dietary guidelines must consist of nutrition experts and leaders in pediatrics, obesity, cardiovascular disease, and public health. Selecting the panelists, however, is a highly politicized process as it is subject to serious high-pressure lobbying from organizations such as the National Dairy Council, United Fresh Fruit and Vegetable Association, Soft Drink Association, American Meat Institute, National Cattlemen's Beef Association, and Wheat Foods Council. The Dietary Guidelines for Americans

> When you increase the intake of foods that are metabolically necessary, you automatically reduce the risk of cancer formation.

2005 continues to reflect the tense interplay of science and the powerful food industry.

With this in mind, the government dietary guidelines set the standards for all federal nutrition programs. This includes school lunches and the food products that many Americans buy. Accurately stated, the guidelines influence how billions of dollars are spent. Hence, even seemingly minor adjustments can help or hurt a particular food industry.

In an ideal world, if the only goal of the government's MyPyramid is to give the public the best possible advice for healthy eating, then it should be based on evidence and not be independent of business interests. But since such is clearly not the case, we must take individual responsibility and become well-informed food and health consumers. Many organizations have taken it upon themselves to educate the public such as the American Cancer Society that repeatedly informed us that if we ate primarily vegetables, fruits, and complex carbohydrates, we just wouldn't have a lot of secondary illnesses such as cancer and heart disease.

The New York Times recently reported that, "A diet low in fat and rich in fruits and vegetables has been found for the first time, to lower blood pressure quickly and as effectively as drugs." Fitness experts, for instance, know that if you base a diet on carbohydrates (60 percent according to that Pyramid) then you must burn more calories with increased activity.

However, the agricultural community was ecstatic over the recommendation! In other words, you just cannot ignore the very real influence of the food industry. After all, anything that affects the food sales of a nation would cause us to understand that it would be naive to think lobbyists of those related interests did not have influence.

When it comes to recommending servings and calories, so much has to be taken into consideration. This is why diets don't work. When it comes to diets, the first question you must ask yourself is, "What are my nutritional needs?" Basing a diet on calories instead of nutritional requirements is a very bizarre concept. Your current health, genetic history, age, sex, activity level, stress level, and climate must all be evaluated in order to get the most from your diet.

By going back to the basics and eating foods as close as possible to their natural state and by slowly eliminating the convenience foods that we have come to rely upon so heavily, you can transform your body first by detoxifying the accumulated poisons and second, by rebuilding it at a cellular, biochemical level, as will be explained in subsequent chapters. Once body transformation has evolved to your satisfaction, you can then ease into a maintenance program by allowing yourself more individual dietary choices.

In place of the USDA Food Guide Pyramid and MyPyramid—old and newly revised—I propose the Body Transformation Food Guide Pyramid. This is a far superior eating plan for weight control and nutritional value, and one that is supported by virtually all those seriously knowledgeable about health and nutrition.

You want *a way of eating for life that is nutritionally dense yet calorie-light*. As we age, caloric needs decline but our nutrient needs increase. The Body Transformation Pyramid is very high in nutritional density but the caloric density per ounce of food is very low.

The goals of this type of eating are simple and direct. From a psychological perspective, this Pyramid provides foods that are truly immunostimulant. This type of diet is the best eating plan for controlling potential heart disease, emotional balance, and for preventing certain types of cancer. This is an immunostimulant diet that offers an anti-aging effect because of its high antioxidant properties. In addition, by adjusting your protein intake, it protects against the loss of muscle tissue as we get older. Our protein needs are very real. Studies indicate that people who go below 50 grams of protein a day, suffer a loss of immune response and muscle strength as well as muscle mass and lean body mass. That's why I don't cut down on protein, but I am not talking about a "high" protein diet. This is a rather moderate amount of protein.

The Body Transformation Pyramid also takes into consideration certain psychological factors, like the element of satiety. Recently, the *European Journal of Clinical Nutrition reported that the top five foods for satiety are potatoes, fish, oatmeal, oranges, and apples* (in this order). These foods are staples of The Body Transformation Pyramid.

Furthermore, people tend to eat large quantities of food. We are not interested in small servings. As we get older, this type of diet allows us to eat a reasonably large amount of food and yet keep the calories and our weight down. Hence, when you consider this Pyramid from a psychological, physiological, nutritional, and caloric point of view, this type of eating comes very close to a diet that prevents illness, stimulates the immune system, increases the energy level, and naturally keeps your weight down.

Although USDA officials claim to have similar goals in mind with their Pyramid, in reality, their creation is absurd. The government's food guide does not differentiate between whole grains and nutritionally depleted (and nutrient depleting once in the body) white flour products, nor, between the dangerous saturated fats and essential fats.

While intentioned to give some kind of nutritional guidelines, the USDA is trying to do it by Harris Poll and by traditional guidelines, which have not really been helpful in the long run. They are not at all taking into account the psychological and behavioral factors—that people are not eating foods in prescribed quantities. Who came up with a half-cup serving anyway? Who eats like this?

Secondly, we must note that the majority of people do not eat natural food. Can you even find whole grain pasta on a restaurant menu, or the supermarket, or Costco? The government nutritionists are not dealing with the realities of day to day life. Bureaucrats and academics brought the USDA Food Guide Pyramid/MyPyramid together and it poorly reflects real life.

It seems that when it comes to our dietary consideration, this is the only area of life where people look to government for how to live. If you go across the board and nature of American society, I don't think the average person believes the government should tell us how to live. But this

> Western societies are over-consuming protein, especially from meat and dairy products.

is the one area of exception. As usual, guidance emanating from Washington is lacking in wisdom.

Most of us who have attempted to control our weight with various diets over the years are basically rather knowledgeable about the nutritional value of various foods. That's why people interested in healthy eating have never had very much respect for the USDA Food Guide Pyramid or MyPyramid. After all, it is just such a diet that made them unhealthy and overweight in the first place.

There is a way of eating to gain greater health, energy and vitality while naturally controlling your weight—it is the Body Transformation Food Guide Pyramid:

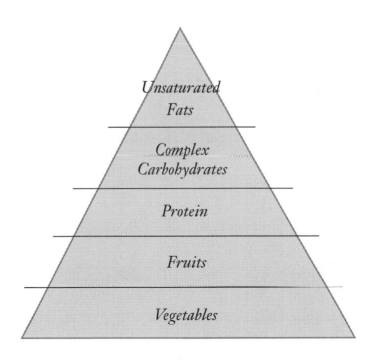

IF IT DOESN'T GROW, DON'T EAT IT

With a great abundance of fruits and vegetables made available to us year round, it's hard to believe that most of us are depriving ourselves of their invaluable goodness. Only nine percent of Americans eat the necessary five or more servings of fruits and vegetables a day—a very low quantity at that. Simple dietary adjustments like drinking a glass of fresh juice in the morning, a salad and vegetables with each meal, a piece of fruit as a snack—the quota can be easily met. At the onset of this decade, the average person was eating barely more than one serving of vegetables and less than one serving of fruit a day!

This is shocking news when you consider how much physical and mental suffering could be avoided by consuming these foods. About 150 studies reviewed by the University of California at Berkeley claimed that eating fruits and vegetables helps prevent various cancers. A Harvard University study determined that women who eat just one serving of certain vegetables or fruits every day have a 40 percent lower risk of stroke and a 22 percent lower risk of heart attack than women who eat very few of these foods. For most cancer sites, people who ate fewer fruits and vegetables were at twice the risk compared with those who consumed more of these foods. It is crucial to remember that a lack of a single serving each day usually adds up to a major deficit in the long run.

Fruits and vegetables are the most effective against cancers that involve epithelial cells, which line the body's organs. This includes cancer of the lung, bladder, cervix, mouth, larynx, throat, esophagus, stomach, pancreas, colon, and rectum.

In addition to their high fiber content, vitamins, minerals, antioxidants, enzymes and other nutrients, scientists are very excited about phytochemicals—the hottest news in nutrition. Phytochemicals (chemicals found in plants) are compounds that give plant food their color, flavor, and also contribute to the plants' self-defense systems. There are hundreds—perhaps thousands—of phytochemicals and each one discovered has a different name, for instance: genistein in soy beans, indoles and isothiocyanates in broccoli, coumarins in tomatoes.

Phytochemicals perform by interfering with the development of cancer at the cellular level. Some of them prevent cancer-causing chemicals from ever developing, while others protect the cells from damage. For instance, carrots and leafy green vegetables can help prevent lung cancer, cruciferous vegetables work against colon cancer, and lettuce and onions guard against stomach cancer.

Certain phytochemicals can prevent the onset of diabetes and others can block infectious diseases by strengthening the immune system. Studies even indicate that phytochemicals may reduce the risk of heart disease.

Phytochemicals are present in all fruits and vegetables, whole grains, beans and many herbs and spices. Scientists agree that it may be one of the best cancer preventers in existence. Experts say that if we are to make gains in preventing cancer, there must be chemopreventive agents that are efficacious and without toxicity. Phytochemicals could be our vitamins of the future.

Top Sources of Phytochemicals:
- Garlic and onions—May block formation of cancer-causing chemicals; lowers cholesterol.
- Hot peppers—Reduce the development of various cancers and prevent toxic substances from attaching to DNA.

The average American diet consists of about 50% carbohydrates, unfortunately, much of it is in the form of white flour and sugar. Such non-foods deplete the body of vitamins, minerals—especially chromium—and lead to diabetes, hypertension, heart disease, anemia, candida, skin disorders, kidney disease, and cancer.

• Carrots, sweet kale, cauliflower, and cantaloupe—Help prevent lung cancer.

• Tomatoes and citrus fruits—Prevent the body's formation of substances that may cause cancer, help prevent blood clots.

• Kale, Brussels sprouts, cabbage, and broccoli—Protect the body against cancer by assisting in the elimination of dangerous toxins.

• Oranges, grapefruits, lemons, and limes—Assist in the production of natural substances that help destroy various cancer-causing substances.

• Raspberries, strawberries, blueberries, and grapes—Aid the body in flushing out toxic chemicals.

When you increase the intake of foods that are metabolically necessary, you automatically reduce the risk of cancer formation. Some people have expressed a concern that consuming the extra dietary fiber found in fruits and vegetables depletes the stores of minerals. However, USDA's Report on Selected Research Projects claims that this is simply not true. While people can suffer from considerable discomfort (indigestion, bloating) while increasing the consumption of fresh fruits and vegetables at first, data strongly suggests that eventually you will tolerate, and soon enjoy and prefer, eating more fresh fruits and vegetables. Others have taken a short cut by juicing, but in terms of phytochemicals, the whole fruit and vegetables are necessary. Juicing removes the pulp—depriving you of fiber and many of the phytochemicals.

THE POWER OF PROTEIN

When the Body Transformation Food Guide Pyramid was shown to various individuals and they were asked if they could live on this way of eating, I was surprised at how many replied, "Not enough protein."

Scientifically, there is great concern that Western societies are over-consuming protein, especially from meat and dairy products. Many of us believe that protein is required for energy, but this assumption is false. Carbohydrates and fats are more readily used for fuel and it is they, not protein that actually nourish the active muscles. Eating large amounts of protein has nothing to do with building muscle or becoming strong and healthy. Just the opposite holds true—too much protein has been associated with diseases such as osteoporosis, heart disease, kidney disease, urinary tract stone formation, and certain cancers.

Protein (amino acids) build the tissue during growth and it is especially necessary during pregnancy, lactation or when an individual is recovering from an illness, surgery, or major burns. Otherwise, an over-consumption of protein can bring on a series of health problems. The incidence of coronary artery disease, for instance, correlates with each country's intake of meat throughout the world. Excess protein is linked to the *diseases of affluence*.

Protein is an essential part of nutrition, second only to water in the body's physical composition. It makes up about 20 percent of our body weight and is a primary component of our muscles, hair, nails, skin, eyes and internal organs—especially the heart and brain. Our immune defense system requires protein, especially for the formation of antibodies that help fight infections.

Protein foods are classified according to their ability to be digested and used by the body. The measurement of this ability is called net protein utilization (NPU) or biological value (BV). Chicken eggs are considered to have the protein of highest known NPU. After eggs, in descending order, are fish, cow's milk and cheese, brown rice, red meat, and poultry. Again, this is not based on protein content but on biological value—how effectively the body utilizes the protein in the food.

When you eat too much protein, the body will have a positive nitrogen balance and growth can occur. Animal protein promotes cancer even more dramatically than does saturated fat. But lowering dietary protein has been shown to reduce tumor growth dramatically. Additionally, those who eat most of their protein from animal sources are more susceptible to heart disease and cancer. It also causes women to mature earlier and early menstruation is linked to an increased risk of reproductive cancers. However, it has also been argued that it is the excessive amount of hormones found in animal meat and dairy products that causes this to occur. When you don't consume enough protein, the body will have a negative balance. About the only people who don't get adequate amounts of protein in their diets are those who eat very little food in general. It is virtually impossible for a basically healthy individual to be protein deficient in Western societies.

Most of our lives, we want to have a neutral nitrogen balance. The amount of protein consumption and protein utilization causes us to move into positive or negative nitrogen balance and to either build more protein or lose some; consequently, this influences body weight, shape, and tone.

Complete Proteins:
Milk, eggs, fish, poultry, and red meats.

Incomplete Proteins:
Grains (low in lysine and isoleucine), legumes (low in tryptophan and methinonine), seeds (low in lysine and isoleucine), and vegetables (most are low in methinoine and isoleucine).

A diet properly balanced for optimal health should derive no more than 15 percent of its calories from protein. Of course, protein requirement should depend on our individual age, weight, and special health concerns. The RDA for protein is 0.36 grams per pound of ideal body weight. This means 44 grams of protein for a 120-pound woman and 56 grams for a 150-pound man. Albeit, many argue that this is still too much. Nevertheless, the typical American woman consumes about 90 grams of protein every day. This isn't hard to do when you consider that a quart of skim milk has 35 grams of protein, three ounces of chicken has 36 grams, and a cup of cottage cheese has 30 grams of protein.

It is especially recommended that we eat fish and seafood as a key source of protein as well as for its beneficial unsaturated oils. Ounce for ounce, most fish is lower in both calories and fat than meat. Fish is also a great source of vitamins (especially

B6 and B12) and minerals like calcium, magnesium, potassium, iron, zinc, selenium, and copper.

The omega-3 fatty acids in fish (especially tuna, salmon, and sardines) has been shown to inhibit the growth of certain cancers and to prevent or relieve the symptoms of inflammatory diseases like arthritis.

Interestingly, some research suggests that the beneficial fats found in fish seem to work only when fish is eaten; fish oil supplements don't appear to provide the same benefits, but the jury is still out on this. Although we consume 50 percent more fish today than we did a decade ago, it still means less than once a week. Ideally, we should be eating six ounces of fish twice a week.

There is a new trend, however, known as "fish farming" that is diminishing its nutritional quality. Almost all catfish, about 90 percent of Atlantic salmon, some 10 percent of chinook, coho and sockeye salmon, and 50 percent of shrimp are raised on these man-made "farms" for at least a part of their lives. On these fish farms, they are fed grains and not smaller fish and plankton. This results in less

Essential fatty acids deficiency is perhaps the most important health problem in America.

omega-3 oils and other nutrients. Therefore, be certain to know the origin of your fish and seafood.

NOT ALL CARBOHYDRATES
ARE CREATED EQUAL

Carbohydrates are an organic molecule; they contain carbon and are derived from living sources. They are produced by photosynthesis in plants and are the primary source of energy in nature's plant foods—fruits, vegetables, grains, legumes and tubers. These foods are vital for the health of your internal organs, the nervous system and the muscles. They are the ideal source of energy since they provide both an immediate and time-released energy source because carbohydrates are digested easily and then steadily metabolized in the bloodstream.

Furthermore, *carbohydrates are necessary for protein regulation and fat metabolism*. Along with the proteins and fats, carbohydrates aid in the fight against infections while promoting growth of body tissues like bones and skin as well as lubricating the joints. Complex carbohydrates are also high in fiber, which helps the body's detoxification process and promotes colon health.

Carbohydrates are classified according to their structure:
MONOSACCHARIDES (simple sugars): honey and fruits.
You should consume a little honey and a lot of fruit.
OLIGOSACCHARIDES (multiple sugars): table sugar and malt sugar.
You should not eat any of these.
POLYSACCHARDIES (starches or complex carbohydrates): vegetables and whole grains. You should eat a lot of these.

Complex carbohydrates are composed of long chains of glucose molecules. They provide a more consistent blood sugar level than the simple sugars, which cause your glucose level in the blood to rise and then drop very quickly. Our modern diet, which leads to so much tissue degeneration and premature aging, is basically composed of refined-flour products and multiple sugars. Although the average American diet consists of about 50 percent carbohydrates, unfortunately, much of it is in the form of white flour and sugar. Such non-foods deplete the body of vitamins, minerals—especially chromium—and lead to diabetes, hypertension, heart disease, anemia, candida, skin disorders, kidney disease, and cancer. We literally have people who are known as "carb addicts"—addicted to refined sugars and suffering with everything from allergies to obesity, not to mention "carbohydrate depression."

Traditionally, people ate the complex carbohydrates such as potatoes, vegetable roots and whole unprocessed grains, which are also a good source of protein, B-vitamins, vitamin-E, iron, magnesium, and some trace minerals such as zinc and copper. All grains are naturally low in fat, but the fat they do contain is the unsaturated beneficial type. It is wise to return to this way of eating: many vegetables, whole grains, and legumes. The only simple sugars we should consume are the "naturally occurring" variety found in fresh fruits.

Our basic, most consumed grains are wheat, rye, oats, corn, barley, buckwheat, couscous, and millet. In the unrefined natural state, they are wholesome and nutritious. But there are also some ancient "supergrains" that have disappeared from our diets and are now once again making a welcomed and much needed comeback.

The ancient grains well deserve the title "the staff of life" because it is for their exceptional nutritional qualities that agricultural entrepreneurs have diligently labored to revive them for today's market.

Amaranth, quinoa, spelt, kamut, and teff should soon be as familiar and as common to us as wheat and corn. Nutritionally, it should replace them in your diet.

For more than 5,000 years, the ancient Incas of South America and the Aztecs of Mexico honored amaranth as "the food of the gods." For centuries, amaranth—a grain that can withstand drought and cold and with its superior nutritional value—was forbidden to be grown. Hernando Cortes, Mexico's Spanish-born conqueror, laid the law that anyone who dared to grow and consume this extraordinary food of life would face the death penalty.

Quinoa, "the mother grain" was named by the Quechua tribe and grows in the Rockies today. The similarities in history and nutritional quality between amaranth and quinoa are striking. Its fluffy texture and distinct flavor and aroma is ideal for pilafs, cold salads and side dishes.

Spelt, possibly the most ancient of cultivated wheats, has grown in Europe for some 9,000 years. Spelt is high in fiber. It's easily digested and is a favorite substitute for those with gluten intolerance and/or wheat allergies.

Kamut was a staple in the Nile 6,000 years ago. The Greeks replaced it with red durum, but in 1970, a Montana farmer reintroduced this terrific grain. Like spelt, it is tolerated by those with wheat allergies.

Teff has been a staple of Ethiopia for thousands of years, most likely due to its ability to withstand rough and lengthy droughts. The world's tiniest grain now grows in Idaho. Its unique distinct flavor and aroma, reminiscent of molasses, and its dense and gelatinous texture make it a favorite for cereals, pancakes, puddings, stews and baked goods. These and other ancient grains are manufactured by Arrowhead Mills, among others, and are available at better health and whole food stores.

Of course, when you increase your level of physical activity by exercising more, you will need to increase your carbohydrate intake—that's the complex variety, as discussed.

FAT: OUR #1
DIETARY DEFICIENCY

The "good fat" that is. Essential fatty acid deficiency is perhaps the most important health problem in America, according the experts at the Boston University Medical Center.

When essential fatty acids are in short supply, *Time* magazine reiterated, the body compensates by substituting other types of fatty acids that have a less supple biochemical structure. As these other compounds replace polyunsaturates, cell membranes become more rigid, leading to progressive hardening of the arterial walls. *The National Cancer Institute* even reported

Olive oil

is quite

possibly our

healthiest

food source.

that diets high in saturated fat lead to lung cancer in non-smoking women and recommended a switch to unsaturated fat.

There are three kinds of dietary fat: monounsaturated, polyunsaturated, and saturated. Saturated fat is most prevalent in the Western diet and a leading cause of clogged arteries and heart disease—our #1 killer of men and women. Unsaturated fat is possibly the least consumed food by Americans and as a result, our health has suffered enormously and needlessly.

Only the polyunsaturated fats are considered *essential*; they cannot be manufactured by the body and thus must be ingested as food. The linoleic acid and linolenic acid found in polyunsaturated fat are crucial to the proper functioning of cell membranes and to the building of potent chemical messengers that regulate everything from blood pressure to the firing of nerves.

Unfortunately, food manufacturers virtually always remove these acids (along with many other healthful nutrients) from foods in order to prolong the packaged food's shelf life. Besides always eating foods as close to their natural state as possible, to increase your intake of linoleic and linolenic acids you must consume more raw seeds, nuts, and green vegetables. Researchers found that people who ate nuts (but avoided peanuts) more than four times a week had a 50 percent lower risk of heart attacks than people who seldom ate nuts. The nuts' high fiber and vitamin-E content, along with the essential fatty acids, help to reduce the artery plaque buildup. However, your intake of saturated fat must be low in order for these benefits to be evident.

Additionally, you must consume the pure (not blended) oils such as corn, safflower, almond, walnut, soybean, fish oils, and especially extra virgin olive oil. Olive oil is quite possibly our healthiest food source. It contains essential fatty acids and has a good variety of vitamins, minerals and some protein. It also contains vitamin-E, vitamin-A, and many of the B-vitamins. Further, olive oil has minerals such as zinc, copper, iron, calcium, magnesium, and phosphorous. It is interesting to note that olive oil seems to do so much more than make food taste good. Research indicates that women who consume at least two tablespoons of pure extra virgin olive oil more than once a day reduce their risk of breast cancer by 25 percent compared to women who don't.

Since 30 percent of our diet (top of the Body Transformation Pyramid) should consist of calories from fat, make it the vital fat, the unsaturated variety for optimal health and longevity.

CHAPTER 5
ARE YOU GOING TO EAT THAT?

While we are mindful of the life-generating properties in food that our bodies require to thrive, we must be aware of some disturbing new developments in food technology that is unsettling to a great number of people. Here, I am specifically talking about food irradiation and genetically engineered foods.

A recent CBS News poll found that, nationwide, 73 percent of those polled oppose food irradiation, and 77 percent say they would not eat irradiated food. However, irradiated food is already a part of your diet and you don't even know it. Soon, it will be a part of our *daily* diet. We are already consuming, albeit unknowingly, many genetically altered foods.

In the ongoing debates about how to best safeguard the nation's food supply against the increase in food-borne disease, one of the tools public health experts are turning to is irradiation. This decades-old technology, which involves exposing *the food we eat to heavy doses of radioactive material*, is being hailed as a quick fix for eradicating dangerous bacteria before food reaches our table. Supporters heartily endorse irradiation as an effective weapon in the food safety arsenal. Skeptics say it's a false solution that only appears to fix the problem of contaminated food without addressing the root cause—sloppy processing practices. They also cite a laundry list of additional concerns, including declines in food quality, potential environmental hazards, uncertainty about its long-term effects on people, and deep distrust that it's the full-spectrum pollution solution it's touted to be.

So what exactly is irradiation? Simply put, when food is irradiated, it is exposed to enough radiation to kill as many microbes as possible while doing as little damage to the food as possible. In theory, it sounds fine. And yet, when food is irradiated, it's shuttled by rail between six-foot thick, steel-reinforced walls to a bunker-like chamber where it's bombarded with gamma rays by either radioactive cobalt-60, cesium-137, x-rays or a beam of high-energy electrons. One shot is powerful: the equivalent of 10,000,000 chest x-rays! *Imagine the food you eat and your family eats, being zapped with the same radioactive materials used at Chernobyl and Three Mile Island.* In the view of many, this is inviting disaster, particularly because substances are being used in industrial buildings that do not use the same precautions employed for nuclear reactors.

In addition to killing certain microorganisms, the process also retards ripening and in some cases, spoilage. To

Imagine the food you eat and your family eats, being zapped with the same radioactive materials used at Chernobyl and Three Mile Island.

extend the shelf life of hamburger or to store strawberries for six weeks instead of two, could mean less waste and more profit— thus its wide appeal to the food industry.

Despite an on-again, off-again flurry of publicity surrounding irradiation, its use on food is nothing new. In 1963, the Food and Drug Administrations (FDA) approved it to control insects in wheat and wheat flour; in 1964 it was OK'd to inhibit the sprouting of white potatoes; in 1983, it was put into service to kill insects and micro-organisms in herbs, spices, and vegetable seasonings; in 1985, it was approved for pork; in 1990, poultry got the go ahead.

The Centers for Disease Control provide this most current list of foods that have been approved for irradiation in the United States. (For meats, separate approval is required both from the FDA and the USDA.)

APPROVAL YEAR	FOOD	DOSE	PURPOSE
1963	Wheat flour	0.2-0.5 kGy	Control of mold
1964	White potatoes	0.05-0.15 kGy	Inhibit sprouting
1986	Pork	0.3-1.0 kGy	Kill Trichina parasites
1986	Fruits and Vegetables	1.0 kGy	Insect control, increase shelf life
1986	Herbs/Spices	30 kGy	Sterilization
1990-FDA	Poultry	3 kGy	Bacterial pathogen reduction
1992-USDA	Poultry	1.5-3.0 kGy	Bacterial pathogen reduction
1997-FDA	Meat	4.5 kGy	Bacterial pathogen reduction
2000-USDA	Meat	4.5 kGy	Bacterial pathogen reduction

Among the latest of developments, as stories about food-borne illness dominate the media, the irradiation industry teamed up with the meat industry to heavily promote the process as a way to assuage public fears of dirty beef. In the summer of 1997, within weeks of the massive 25 million-pound Hudson Meats recall of contaminated ground beef, a spate of articles on irradiation appeared in major U.S. newspapers with virtually the same message: Irradiation is the answer to worries about food safety.

Cast as Robocop, a high-tech protector designed to restore order to a food supply gone haywire, irradiation has won over a rainbow coalition of supporters in the food production and public health communities. An impressive array of organizations, ranging from the World Health Organization (WHO), the American Medical Association (AMA), and the Council of State and Territorial Epidemiologists, to a number of food trade associations, including the United Fresh Fruit and Vegetable Association, is making the push for irradiation—although all agree it is only part of the answer. Other food safety groups, such as Safe Tables Our Priority (STOP) and Center for Science in the Public Interest (CSPI), which have not come out in support of irradiation, report pressure from the irradiation industry to do so.

Opponents warn that far from being the savior of the nation's food supply, irradiation is actually a Pandora's Box of health and environmental woes we haven't even begun to realize. Widespread use is a decision that will come back to haunt us, many believe. One can logically conclude that food irradiation is not the cure its advocates want us to believe it is, but instead allows the causes of meat contamination to flourish while giving the false appearance that the problem is being solved. Instead of being forced to clean up inhumane, filthy and sloppy processing facilities, corporations can continue the practices that lead to contamination and simply irradiate the fecal-contaminated meat products that should have been discarded in the first place.

Another persuasive argument against irradiation is a marked decline in the food quality. Indeed, according to WHO's report, "Safety and Nutrition Adequacy of Irradiated Food" considered the definitive analysis of irradiation's effects on food and the document on which irradiation supporters base their arguments—the process saps food of crucial vitamins and minerals. These include vitamins A, B2, B6, B12, C, E, K, folic acid, and thiamine.

Equating vitamin losses in irradiated foods to those in products that are canned, heated or processed in other ways, the WHO report states the impact of such nutritional losses depends on how much of a particular food is eaten. "As long as such foods constitute only a small fraction of the daily food consumption, concern is unwarranted, especially when irradiation is limited to items such as spices, which do not contribute to the vitamin supply," they claim.

But while vitamin loss in say, oregano, may be inconsequential, nutrient depletion could become a much larger mainstay of our diet. One study cited in the WHO report showed 50 percent less vitamin-C in irradiated potatoes. Another study cited in the same report, found that thiamine levels in irradiated codfish were down a full 50 percent as well. Such things are of particular concern to those who maintain that we don't know what the long-term effects of such deficiencies will have on people who eat large amounts of irradiated food. We ought to demand that every food that is irradiated be tested pre- and post-irradiation as well as tested after it is cooked, and that information about nutrition depletion be put on the label so consumers can choose whether to eat it or not.

The World Health Organization says that the introduction of irradiated foods into the food supply is likely to be gradual and to extend over a long period, providing ample time for elevation. In other words, in this shocking scenario, we'll just figure it out as we go; we the consumers will be the test animals.

Even more worrisome, irradiation opponents contend, is that "sanitizing" food with radioactive material damages the product's basic molecular structure, forming free radicals (known to contribute to cancer and heart disease among many other problems) within the food, which then enter our bodies when we consume it. These free radicals, in turn, react to form small amounts of chemical substances such as formaldehyde, formic acid, quinones, and carcinogen benzene, all of which are known to be hazardous to our health. In addition, completely new chemicals called unique radiolytic products, which have not been identified nor tested for toxicity, are formed.

There's no question that irradiation creates free radicals—even proponents of irradiation readily admit this fact. The

> We ought to demand that every food that is irradiated be tested pre- and post-irradiation as well as tested after it is cooked, and that information about nutrition depletion be put on the label so consumers can choose whether to eat it or not.

question is the extent to which they do harm in the body. Irradiation proponents argue that ordinary cooking methods (like boiling) create their own cache of free radicals. But still unanswered is the cumulative effect of eating cooked irradiated foods.

Proponents also point to numerous studies done on test animals fed irradiated foods to show that levels of free radicals generated by irradiation are minuscule, certainly not enough to assault human health. Other scientists insist that the animal studies done by the FDA on irradiation are seriously flawed—in a word, sloppy. The only way to test the effects of irradiation is not to give animals whole foods, but to extract the potentially toxic products of irradiation and to then use standard methods of testing for carcinogenicity, which involves using highly concentrated doses (about 100 times higher than what humans would ingest) to make up for the small population sample.

The FDA had not conducted such tests as they are too expensive. Until such fundamental studies are undertaken, there's little scientific basis for accepting the industry's assurances of safety. More distressing is that the scientific literature contains numerous animal studies, which demonstrate that consumption of irradiated food creates mutations that result in mutated cells known as polyploidy. The WHO committee responsible for drafting the irradiation report examined these studies and blithely dismissed the findings stating, "No significance can be attributed to polyploidy in terms of any *specific* disease."

Critics say this response is arbitrary and capricious. This WHO committee had a singular lack of expertise in public health, preventive medicine and cancer research. These are genetic mutations. Any mutation is dangerous. It may precede cancer. It indicates abnormalities in the metabolic processes and gene changes have the potential to be transmitted.

Based on what scientists know we cannot treat the production of polyploidy cells that dismissively. The issue of abnormalities will not be resolved until studies are done in which a selected group is fed irradiated foods as a significant part of their diet for three months. It may have negative results but it has to be done.

What about irradiation and the environment? With the prospect of irradiation facilities gearing up nationwide—the United States currently has about 100, and 350 more are reportedly being planned—safety for the environment, facility workers as well as people who live nearby is a looming issue.

Internationally, the Nuclear Regulatory Commission has recorded 54 accidents at 132 irradiation facilities since 1974. More current data has been difficult to obtain. A facility in Dickerson, Maryland, that irradiates medical supplies (a long-standing and accepted practice) was cited by the Maryland Department of the Environment for having "failed to maintain radiation exposures to members of the public living near the plant to levels as low as reasonably achievable." Violations included radioactive cobalt-60 particles found in private residential properties near the plant and citations for failing to clean up contaminated soil in public areas.

Many experts worry about the increased potential for accidents that may result simply from transporting radioactive material like cobalt-60 and cesium-137, if more irradiation facilities open around the country. Indeed, to irradiate even just the fruits produced in Fresno, CA, alone would require 57 plants!

Irradiation is not sterilization, a common misunderstanding. At approved doses, the process kills most relatively large organisms including most bacteria, but it's unable to destroy viruses, which are smaller and more resistant. But some microorganisms, such as the hardy Clostridium botulinum and Clostridium perfringens, which can contaminate both meat and vegetables, can survive irradiation in enough numbers to trigger illness. In the vacuum-packaging hamburger would require to prevent it from turning brown, these oxygen-hating bacteria could, if present, produce a disease-causing toxin. According to meat industry researchers, once the natural balance between good and bad bacteria has been destroyed, any contamination of the product that occurs after it's been irradiated, say, at the supermarket or even your favorite restaurant, creates the potential for bacteria growth to reach dangerous levels.

And through irradiation, we may be inadvertently creating even more deadly pathogens. In 1995, *New Science* magazine reported that some bacteria could actually survive levels of irradiation thousands of times greater than those that would kill humans. This raises the alarming possibility that irradiation could be fostering superstrains of irradiation-resistant bacteria, a situation that's reminiscent of the supergerms bred by overuse of antibiotics.

The end result of irradiation is that consumers would still have to tread cautiously with irradiated products, essentially treating them the same way as non-irradiated products—washing hands and preparation surfaces after handling them and cooking everything thoroughly. So, here's the big question: What then has ultimately been achieved except more processing, more costs, and potential risk?

Although the industry, and oddly enough, the medical association, has been pushing for food irradiation, the public has thus far stood firmly against it. However, we know that it's only a matter of time before the general public is worn down in its resistance. On April 29, 2004 an article and a perspective piece appeared in the New England Journal of Medicine, both making a plea to doctors across America and other health care providers to push for more irradiation of foods in order to help kill potentially deadly germs. The article claims about 76 million cases of food-borne illness, resulting in more than 325,000 hospitalizations and 5,000 deaths occur annually in the United States The Centers for Disease Control and Prevention state that this rate could be reduced from 76,000,000 to 75,100,000 cases and we would have 352 fewer deaths.

Currently, the United States produces eight billion pounds of ground beef annually and 0.32 percent of it is contaminated with the E.coli bacterium.

In response to this, the national director of the Organic Consumers Association has pointed out that, "If we had a system comparable to that of northern Europe with strict regulations and zero tolerance for contaminants, we wouldn't be having the problem in the first place. Let's follow that line of thinking rather than just assume we've got a horrible situation getting worse that we can only solve with a problematic technology."

Nevertheless, the push is on for irradiation and it is catching on, even if very slowly at present. Proponents have publicly argued that at present, the market for irradiated food is small and could be boosted if there was a mandate to serve it in government-sponsored nutrition programs such as schools, day care centers, and so forth.

Perhaps by coincidence, the 2002 farm bill required the USDA to offer irradiated beef to schools, even though no one has asked for it. The USDA now offers (as of January 2004) irradiated ground beef to schools all across America—about 27 million children. And soon, the U.S. Food and Drug

Administration may authorize irradiation of cold cuts and processed meats as well.

Fortunately, parents have taken notice and started calling schools to tell them that their children will be brown bagging their lunches if this happens. *The New York Times* has reported that critics claim that not enough studies have been done to prove irradiated beef is safe; that in fact some studies have shown that it may promote cancer and that it should not be given to children until the concerns are met.

Julie Korenstein, a member of the Los Angeles school board introduced a resolution that the board passed in September 2003, banning all irradiated foods from schools for five years. "I was not particularly enamored of using 750,000 children as guinea pigs," Korenstein was reported as saying.

The Organic Consumers Association reported that the Agriculture Department sent a letter and information brochure to school superintendents urging them to "engage in an educational effort of food irradiation before ordering irradiated product." Aware of the uphill battle for acceptance, the brochure offered assurance about the safety of irradiation and noted that it had been endorsed by several health organizations, including the FDA and CDC. It said irradiation "can increase the safety of the food supply and help protect consumers from food-borne illness." But it also said that it was not a substitute for good sanitation or safe food handling.

About the same time, in another instance, yet another brochure was produced as part of a pilot education program in three Minnesota school districts. But there were problems. It has been stated that "the material was more promotional than informational." Thus far, none of the districts that participated in these irradiation education pilots had bought any irradiated beef. Perhaps people are being frightened by the mere terminology. The irradiation industry, with the help of U.S. Senator Tom Harkin (D-Ia), is persuading government to have irradiated products be labeled with the more user-friendly term "cold pasteurization."

Further, in this age of "terrorism," there is yet another problem to consider according to a Nobel Peace Prize nominee, Helen Caldicott. A potential terrorist strike against the irradiation plant would be devastating. Caldicott, founder of the Nuclear Policy Institute in Washington, D.C., says we have a problem because of "sloppy, inefficient factory farms" and do not need to apply enough radiation to our food to kill a human being in order to deal with potentially contaminated food. Besides the dangers of eating food exposed to radiation, having a facility such as the one in Milford Township, where she protested on November 22, 2004, is inherently dangerous. "Because the cobalt-60 must remain cold," she said, "a terrorist wouldn't even need a bomb or a gun. All they would have to do is fly or drive into a cooling pond; that would cause the release of 30 times the amount of radiation in a single rod."

About 60% of our processed foods now have some genetically engineered ingredients in them.

If not irradiation, then what? After the 1993 outbreak of E. coli 1057 poisonings from undercooked hamburgers sold by the fast food chain *Jack in the Box*, public health industry officials and agricultural experts met at Washington State University in Pullman to develop effective protocols for controlling E. coli 1057. Among their recommendations: revamped processing for both meat and produce, stricter regulation at all check points; improved certification of food handlers, identification of potential contamination hazards, implementation of quality assurance programs, and consumer education. It's interesting to note that irradiation rated 13th on their list.

As health-conscious consumers, we must also rethink our own food expectations for we share some of the responsibility for what fosters food-borne illness, namely consumer demand for novelty, year-round availability, convenience and cheap food. Accustomed as we are to having our favorite fruits and vegetables always available, it can be difficult to remember that there is a season for everything. It's worth noting that no one gets sick from eating locally grown raspberries in season.

Looking for a quick fix to the complex problem of a polluted food supply is tempting. But irradiation opens the door to more serious concerns about nutritional losses, resistant new strains of bacteria, molecular changes, and environmental challenges—all with potentially serious long-term consequences.

While *food irradiation is the embalming of our diet*, consider what critics are calling *Frankenfood*, or as it is officially known, genetically engineered foods. Would you eat a potato genetically engineered to contain its own pesticide? How about a strawberry that fends off frost courtesy of flounder genes? Or a juicy E. coli-resistant hamburger?

Sound appetizing? If you think these foods are sci-fi fantasy, think again. In fact, such foods are already a regular part of your diet. About 60 percent of our processed foods now have some genetically engineered ingredients in them. While you may never taste genetically engineered ingredients in your corn-flakes, frozen waffles, or soy burgers, chances are good that they're there.

Approximately 70 percent of the foods we eat *could* contain genetically engineered compounds and the number is growing.

"Could?" you ask? The food industry does not want you to know this little secret. When it comes to genetically modified (GM) food, Europeans at least, aren't biting. But *while American companies must label GM foods to sell it in Europe, no law requires them to give American consumers the same information.*

The biotech industry boasts that 90 percent to 95 percent of plant life may be genetically modified in the next five years. Indeed, acreage planted with genetically modified crops increased five-fold in just one year. Whether this rapid growth is something to rejoice in or fear is not entirely clear. The immediate problem is that you can't know for sure if you're eating these foods because the government does not require labeling.

This "brave new world" of genetic engineering allows scientists to pick desired genes from one organism—say, a virus, bacteria or even an animal—and insert them into a completely different life form such as corn or a tomato plant. Up until now, scientists have been using the technology to create plants that can fight crippling viruses to produce crops that are resistant to pests and herbicides and to make food last longer. On the horizon is a plethora of intriguing possibilities—for example: inserting oral vaccines and vitamins into food or even altering its fat content.

This is, of course, dabbling in DNA. This is done by splicing a desirable gene from one plant, animal, or microorganism into DNA in the hopes that the new organism will incorporate the specific trait expressed by that gene. Scientists call the result of these gene transfers "recombinant DNA" (rDNA) and the foods it creates "transgenic" foods or genetically modified (GM) food. The major players in the gene game are DuPont, Monsanto, and Novartis.

There's no question the new technology alters DNA, the genetic blueprint of life. But from a safety and moral point, one must consider the wisdom of transferring genes from one species to another.

Many people consider it a revolution in the way we grow our food. The reason that many of us haven't heard much about it is that after consultation with other experts in the field, the FDA decided in 1992 that genetic engineering isn't a revolution at all. In fact, the FDA considers it not substantially different from the kind of conventional crop breeding that farmers have been doing for centuries. After all, we eat nectarines (bred from peaches), tangelos (tangerines crossed with grapefruits), and corn (crossbred from many different varieties) with no problem. These are foods crossbred from related genes—in other words, from other fruits and vegetables.

Surprisingly, the FDA considers inserting an animal gene into a plant—a fish gene into a tomato, for instance—to be so similar that it hasn't changed its policy since 1992. This means that, as with non-genetically engineered foods, the FDA doesn't require safety testing before these products go to the market. Unfortunately, for the consumer, as I already stated, you won't be told what you're eating.

So who makes sure these food *products* are safe? The FDA relies on the manufacturer for that. But while the agency offers guidance and strongly encourages the manufacturers "for their own best interest" to conduct tests and to consult with the FDA on their new genetic combinations, the bottom line is that companies don't have to do any of it if they don't want to. So far, they have all complied, but there's no governing body to which they're held accountable. And there's no way to know for certain what the long-term effect of GE foods will be.

The lack of an official overseer and required safety testing troubles many scientists who see a big difference between traditional breeding of close relatives on the farm and the new technique of combining genes from totally different species in the laboratory. It's completely artificial. It snips our genes and moves them via test tubes into other organisms. There are those who worry that scientists won't be alerted to any risks posed by genetic engineering because they begin with the *presumption* that there aren't going to be any problems!

But we must consider the risks. Just as no one has concrete proof that genetically engineered foods on the market today are unsafe to eat; there is no proof that they are safe either. On one side, we have the presumption that they ought to be okay, on the other, we have reasoning that some might be okay, as well as a collection of relatively small, often preliminary experiments that suggest that they may not be. Here are some of the most troubling questions that those studies raise about GE foods:

Will these foods contain hidden allergy-producing substances?
Although most of us know what foods trigger our particular allergies and how to avoid them, there's concern that if

genes from another organism can be inserted into a plant, we will no longer be able to recognize those allergy-causing foods.

In the mid-90s, a biotech seed company tried putting Brazil nut genes in soybeans to boost their nutritional value. In a small study, researchers discovered that human volunteers who were allergic to Brazil nuts experienced strong allergic reactions to extracts of the soybeans. The company halted its plans.

Although the FDA requires companies to label known allergens and to investigate suspected ones, some scientists worry about the potential allergens that we don't recognize—such as proteins that come from soil bacteria, not from food. (Most allergens are proteins.) How do you know whether that bacteria, if it were eaten in the same quantities that you eat a food, such as shrimp, would cause allergies or not? Currently, there is simply no adequate way to test that.

Will these foods increase resistance to antibiotics?

Some scientists have suggested that the process of genetic engineering could accelerate antibiotic resistance in humans. When genetic engineers transfer a gene from one life form to another, they also include a "marker" gene that confers antibiotic resistance. This helps them identify and select the cells that have successfully taken up the gene of interest. Some worry that ingesting these genes could not only reduce the effectiveness of a dose of antibiotics, but also eventually render antibiotics virtually powerless to fight some of our most serious infections.

Will genetic engineering change the nutritional value of food?

When soybeans that were genetically engineered to resist the weed killer Roundup (known as "Roundup Ready" soybeans), it was discovered that genetic engineering just might change the nutritional value. Roundup Ready soybeans showed as much as a 20 percent drop in valuable phytoestrogens, which evidence has shown may be beneficial in fighting osteoporosis and heart disease.

Although more testing needs to be done, the implications are significant given that 50 percent of the soybean crop in the United States is Roundup Ready. Beyond soybeans, without more extensive testing, we may not be able to anticipate such nutritional changes in other foods. When such *foods* are so widely spread among the unsuspecting public and a serious health issue arises in the future as a result, there will be no control sample of the population to be found to conduct the appropriate studies in the future.

Will genetic engineering make food toxic?

When a group of rats were fed GE potatoes, they showed signs of intestinal changes. Heated debate ensued about whether the process could make foods toxic. In the study, published in the British medical journal *The Lancet*, researchers suggested that inserting the genetic engineering material "package" to help make potatoes resistant to pets is what caused a thickening of the rats' guts and dramatic changes in their organ weights.

> This "brave new world" of genetic engineering allows scientists to pick desired genes from one organism— say, a virus, bacteria or even an animal —and insert them into a completely different life form such as corn or a tomato plant.

Transferring a gene from one species into another may result in unpredictable changes.

Can the unexpected happen?

It already has. Despite claims that genetic engineering is more "precise" than traditional breeding, some experiments have gone awry and very unexpected results have turned up. They range from a GE soil microbe that unexpectedly killed wheat plants to a field of petunias genetically engineered to turn white that instead bloomed in a riot of colors.

Although scientists caught these potential problems before the products were on the market, that may not always be the case as suggested by a controversial study at Cornell University. This study showed that monarch butterfly larvae died after eating milkweed dusted with GE corn pollen containing a pesticide. The study itself has since been criticized and its ecological implications widely debated, but it reinforced the concern that genetically engineered food may present ripple effects that we can't completely anticipate—or *reverse*.

To eat or not to eat. The idea that we are currently growing and eating genetically engineered food without realizing it and without solid evidence of what the ultimate health and environmental effect, if any, might be, should not sit well with any reasonable person especially those of us who wish to exercise some measure of control over our own well being. So what can you do if you are concerned?

Eat organic. Most places now have whole foods stores and farmer's markets that provide a wide variety of organic foods. This is as good a guarantee as you can get that a product is chemical-free and not genetically altered.

Demand labeling. There needs to be legislation. The Genetically Engineered Food Right to Know Act was debated before Congress. It would require both the FDA and the USDA to label all foods that are genetically engineered or made from genetically engineered ingredients; this has not yet happened. Contact your representative to express your opinion.

Speak your mind. A number of federal regulatory agencies are currently reconsidering their stance on genetically engineered foods. A few years ago, the FDA held a series of three public meetings to "take the pulse of the American public on the issue of genetically engineered foods." Based on comments from these meetings, the agency is reviewing its policy.

At the end of the day, answers are in short supply. When I began research of this topic, I had hoped to give you a handy list of foods that contained genetically engineered ingredients so that you could make your own choices. Was I naive! Product lists can give examples, but the bottom line is that in the processed-foods aisle of your grocery store, most foods are likely to contain ingredients that come from genetically engineered organisms.

On the horizon is a plethora of intriguing possibilities— for example: inserting oral vaccines and vitamins into food or even altering its fat content.

That's because most processed foods contain something that comes from corn or soy—all the more reason to avoid processed foods.

Happily, if you're talking about organic produce, you're not likely to encounter genetically engineered food. There are two grocery store chains that have taken a pledge to eliminate genetically engineered ingredients from their store brands: Whole Foods Market, Inc. (including Fresh Fields, Bread & Citrus, Bread of Life, and Wellspring Grocery) and Wild Oats Markets, Inc. (including Alfalfa's Market, Oasis Fine Foods, Sunshine Grocery, Ideal Market, and Wild Oats Community Market).

Around the world, the U.S. appears to be the Lone Ranger among large countries in embracing biotech. Most other countries believe exporters of GM crops should identify which foods may contain rDNA, although the United States and five smaller countries blocked this proposal at a recent global conference, as it would seriously limit the export market for GM foods.

In Canada, the milk-producing hormones rBST is banned and GM crops are limited as to where they can be planted. In Britain, Prince Charles had taken a very public stance against GM foods, even encouraging consumers to boycott imported GM foods. Several countries are trying to ban GM foods altogether.

Even the most ardent opponents of biotech concede GM foods are likely here to stay. The battle now is over the issue of choice. But having a choice requires knowledge and labeling. So, while we are on a weight-loss and optimal health mission—so diligently avoiding simple carbohydrates, bad fats and sugar in general, and doing everything in our power to obtain and maintain high energy and vitality, we simply *must* be aware of the unseen forces that can rob us of optimal health—our birthright.

CHAPTER 6
USE IT OR LOSE IT

How can we achieve total body fitness? Many people who exercise regularly do not actually possess total body fitness. There are many weight lifters that can bench-press 400 pounds, but they cannot walk around the block without huffing and puffing! There are aerobics fanatics who cannot do ten push-ups.

To be physically fit, you must possess the following: cardiovascular fitness (endurance), muscular fitness (strength), flexibility, co-ordination, speed, agility, and mobility.

A cross-training program that allows you to engage in various activities for greater flexibility, muscle fitness, and endurance shapes your physical destiny. Flexibility concerns the movement of joints. It allows you to do everything from performing daily tasks to engaging in sports with greater ease. Muscular strength allows you to get through the day with greater ease and less fatigue. Strong muscles make for a better posture and a strong heart and a healthy circulatory system, which provides the muscles with more oxygen. This will make you feel alert, vigorous, and energetically younger.

If you exercise regularly but limit yourself to a repetitive regimen, you are getting health benefits but not total body conditioning. It's sort of like being on a healthy diet but eating the very same foods day in and day out. Eventually, you will develop deficiencies. A balanced exercise program is just as important as a balanced diet for optimal health.

A regular exercise program provides so many benefits that I can't imagine anyone living without it. In a very short amount of time, you will feel more relaxed, more alert, energy will be increased, you will require less sleep, and achieve a deeper level of sleep at night. You will not slump around all day, body fat will go down, and your self-esteem will go up. In a nutshell, you will feel really good about yourself. So why aren't more of us working out regularly?

Only about eight percent of the American population exercises adequately enough to maintain *minimal* cardiovascular fitness. It is no wonder that so many Americans are ill and obese. Other developed nations like Britain are just as badly off. The Royal College of Physicians issued a report stating that the levels of habitual physical activity in the general British population are so low that merely walking for a short time at a normal pace may be more than many people can comfortably tolerate!

When other nations adapt American lifestyles, they fall prey to our maladies as well. For example, by the age of 40, half of the British men and three-quarters of all women spend the vast majority of their waking lives in chairs. At the age of 12 years, 70 percent of us engaged in vigorous physical activity. But by age 21, this activity falls to 30 percent for women, and continues to decline as we get older.

The British Heart Foundation reported that less than one in five British people take enough exercise to benefit their hearts. *In sedentary people, muscles actually start wasting away from the mid-20s, after which about half a pound of muscle is traded every year for half a pound of fat.* The underside changes in blood fat chemistry that eventually results in heart disease can even be found in the arteries of inactive primary school children.

A woman reaches her physical maturity by the age of 18 or 19. If she is sedentary, that's when aging begins to creep in on her. The heart loses its ability to pump blood at a rate of one percent every single year past physical maturity. Additionally, the chest wall stiffens and the body is less able to take in oxygen. Muscles become weaker, the metabolism slows down, bones lose calcium, and nerve impulses travel slowly.

If you are sedentary, your blood vessels will be constricted by some 30 percent, which will naturally affect your heart. By the age of 30, you will lose nearly five percent of your muscle fibers. By the age of 60, up to 30 percent of your muscles will be replaced by fat. Worse yet, the blood flow from arms to legs can slow down by up to 60 percent. Eventually, your body's flexibility and bone mass deteriorate. All of this doesn't occur instantly, but by the time you are 40, ALL will be evident! Before you realize it, life as you once knew it, is over.

The U.S. Centers for Disease Control report that *inadequate exercise has about the same affect on the body as smoking a pack of cigarettes every day. They further claim that inactivity is the single most dangerous risk factor in heart disease—greater than high blood pressure, cholesterol, or smoking.* In fact, physically fit people who smoked, had elevated blood pressure, and/or high cholesterol levels lived longer than the sedentary people with none of these risk factors, according to the Cooper Institute for Aerobics in Dallas.

The Journal of the American Medical Association reported that being a couch potato is as unhealthy as smoking. This study tracked more than 32,000 people for nearly a decade and found that inactivity is comparable to such heart disease risk factors as smoking, high blood pressure, and elevated cholesterol levels. Those who were even moderately fit had at least a 17 percent lower death rate than those in the low-fitness groups. Indeed, physically fit smokers are better off than sedentary non-smokers!

Many people who exercise regularly do not actually possess total body fitness.

Even though exercise and the heart have been closely correlated for quite some time, evidence clearly shows that people are far more disciplined about taking medication over the long term than they are about exercising. Research at the University of California has revealed that *exercise is just as effective as drugs in lowering elevated blood pressure*—and with a great many other benefits and none of the side effects. More than 60 million people have high blood pressure that can be greatly managed without the use of drugs.

In Britain, where most of the population is chronically inactive, 65 percent of all women over the age of 50 have above normal blood pressure. A mind-boggling 90 percent have elevated cholesterol levels, which can lead to heart disease. It has been concluded that regular dynamic exercise of moderate intensity can reduce the incidence of coronary events and deaths from heart disease by more than 50 percent. The British Medical Journal reported that the impressive contribution of exercise as prevention should not be underestimated.

Obviously, not just a preventive measure, exercise is being prescribed by type, intensity, and duration. And with good reason. We have strayed far from our biological blueprint and are now paying the price with needless mental and physical suffering. This is all too apparent in the United States. The modern American way of life has resulted in brain chemistry changes in the majority of sedentary people, leading to extraordinary rates of various levels of depression. Scientists have determined that *the rate of depression in the United States has increased more than 20-fold since 1950.* It is estimated that before this decade is over, 50 percent of the American population will be diagnosed with some type of mental disorder.

Research has also shown that depression is directly associated with recreational drug use and television-watching time. Those who regularly participate in sports, however, rarely have episodes of depression. Therefore, depression and a lack of physical activity appear extremely well linked. Recently, it has been documented that depression is the single most definitive personality factor that distinguishes physically active people from sedentary middle-aged American men. On the other hand, it has been consistently found that healthy inactive adults show significant decreases in depression after they begin to exercise.

Even if one must rely on psychotherapy to resolve emotional problems, exercise has been proven a valuable adjunct. It is a much preferred substitute for antidepressants, tranquilizers, sleeping pills, and other drugs. After all, exercise and antidepressant drugs produce similar effects on the brain neuro-transmitter systems, which regulate mood, and both usually reduce symptoms.

However, biochemical treatments don't always work—not to mention the side effects, which can include (depending on the drug) drowsiness, loss of sexual function, skin rashes, and constipation. Exercise, on the other hand, not only lifts most depressions, or better yet, prevents depression from coming on in the first place, it improves the areas that the drugs oppress. The American Psychological Association reported that, "Running should be viewed as a wonder drug, analogous to penicillin, morphine, and the tricyclics."

Exercise is most effective in the reduction of stress and depression when it involves prolonged, rhythmic and controlled breathing. Long-distance runners refer to the exercise-induced "runner's high." This is the result of their bodies producing endorphins, which are natural opiates. Endorphins have been proven to block pain and to create a feeling of well being. Those who exercise regularly show a measurable, reproducible increase in their blood levels of endorphins. Exercise may also favorably alter brain levels of

Only about 8% of the American population exercises adequately enough to maintain *minimal* cardiovascular fitness.

various neurotransmitters such as norepinephrine, serotonin, and dopamine.

Scientists have discovered that physically active people improve their brain function and the nervous system, as much as their circulatory systems. An exceptional medical review conducted by Stanford University that scrutinized more than 80 studies concluded that 70 percent of them revealed the important gains to be made in mental health when a person becomes physically fit. Many experts today theorize that *the brain may be similar to muscles in that it too could lose its capabilities when not used.*

In fact, the very latest research indicates that physical activity improves the ability of the brain to function and process information. Studies have shown that exercise increases the brain processing speed of older adults and improves the intelligence of children. Aerobic exercise fuels the brain with more nutrients, and skill-based exercise increases the number of synapses, or connections, which is believed to make the brain able to process information. In animal studies, the rats that had exercised on the treadmill had a greater density of blood vessels in the brain than did either the acrobatic or inactive animals.

Thus, regular exercise can improve the speed with which the brain processes information. Aerobic exercise increases the amount of certain brain chemicals that stimulate the growth of nerve cells. Reports such as these allow us to conclude that *declines associated with getting older are actually the result of a decline in physical activity.* Reduced mental functioning often attributed to aging, may very well be the result of a sedentary lifestyle and NOT age.

Very few of us get anywhere near adequate exercise indeed. Even though many think that America is a nation of fitness fanatics, trends for obesity and physical inactivity in the U.S. have not improved, according to the NIH conference on this issue. Even if we participate in it enthusiastically for a while, dropout rates are enormously high. For instance, less than 12 percent of women maintain a fitness routine for more than a year. Yet, when it comes to the human body, the worst thing you can do to it is nothing at all. Unlike most machines, *the body actually falls apart from lack of use, not overuse.*

The "disease syndrome" is a new term coined by health practitioners. It describes succinctly how our sophisticated physical system falls pray to various unnatural conditions because of a sedentary lifestyle. Most of the illnesses we associate with the aging process are brought on by our lack of respect for our bodies. Most cases of heart disease, arthritis, mental disorders, and so on, are not a result of misfortune but of poor management.

Fortunately, such a sad state of affairs cannot only be arrested but reversed. Unfortunately, the relevant question most people ask is, "How little physical activity must I carry out in order to be healthy?" Instead of, "How much physical activity can I do to achieve optimal health?"

Nevertheless, the body responds appreciatively to use and it won't be long before it lets you know just how grateful it really is. In a matter of weeks, your resting heart rate will become lower, your fat will begin turning into muscle, your bones will become stronger and you will sleep better, for starters.

In Great Britain, a Royal College of Physicians report claims that following a mere eight weeks of regular exercise, sufficient and demonstrable biochemical adaptations take place. A little exercise is better than none, while more is better than a little. The consensus is that every single adult should accumulate

30 minutes or more of moderate-intensity physical activity over preferably every day of the week.

One condition that is not usually referred to as a disease but is considered as such by many experts, is obesity—definitely a lifestyle factor and a very dangerous one at that. Dieting has become a multi-billion dollar business, with diet foods and drinks alone exceeding $32 billion in the United States— not to mention the money expended on commercial diet plans, clinics, health spas, and all the other things that comprise the weight-loss industry. Today, there are more than 30,000 different diets, all claiming to be the sure-fire way to lose weight and keep it off. A huge number of people—a quarter of the American population in fact—are dieting at any given time. But very few of them actually lose weight, and if they do, even fewer manage to keep it off for long.

A sedentary lifestyle is believed to be one of the key reasons for such an epidemic of obesity. The combination of sedentary work, television watching, and the consumption of high-calorie junk food is lethal. The average person eats about 40 tons of food in a lifetime, including more than 150 pounds of sugar a year. A person may actually be eating fewer calories yet be far more overweight than someone else. Studies show that in such cases, physical activity is the determining factor.

The problem with being overweight is that it often leads to many other potential health problems, such as high levels of cholesterol in the blood, as I've already mentioned. Scientists have shown that exercise lowers LDL cholesterol (the bad kind) and increases HDL cholesterol (the good kind), particularly in combination with weight loss.

Recently, researchers from around the world have been examining the association between exercise and various types of

In sedentary people, muscles actually start wasting away from the mid-20s, after which about half a pound of muscle is traded every year for half a pound of fat.

cancer. Colon cancer—the most common cancer in the U.S. and the second most common cancer in the United Kingdom, which in England and Wales affects one in every 100,000 people between the ages of 40 and 45, and one in every 250 people after 80 years of age—is the first for which scientists have been able to determine a serious link. Researchers at Harvard University scrutinized the cancer history of 17,000 men for up to 23 years and discovered that those who were moderately to highly physically active had a 50 percent lower risk of colon cancer than those who participated in minimal amounts of physical activity. "Moderately active" is defined as the burning of more than 1,000 calories per week in recreational activity. This can translate into jogging or playing tennis two hours a week or simply walking ten miles a week. And yet, most people choose not to do even this little bit.

This led the Surgeon General's first ever report on physical activity and health. President Clinton's Health and Human Services then Secretary, Donna Shalala commissioned it. "This report is nothing else than a national call to action," she stated. *"Physical inactivity is a serious nationwide public health problem."*

The Surgeon General's report emphasizes two important findings. First, demonstrated health benefits occur at a "moderate" level of activity—a level sufficient to expend about a 150 calories of energy per day or 1,000 calories per week (e.g., walking briskly for 30 minutes a day). Second, although physical activity does not need to be vigorous to provide health benefits, the amount of health benefit is directly related to the amount of regular physical activity. These conclusions suggest, according to the Journal of the American Medical Association, a flexible approach to increasing physical activity. Because a moderate amount of exercise can be achieved in various ways and must be sustained throughout life to produce benefits, persons unable or unwilling to adhere to a structured exercise program can incorporate into their daily lives physical activity appropriate to their personal preferences and life circumstances.

Examples of moderate activity include playing volleyball for 45 minutes, raking the leaves for 30 minutes, swimming laps for 20 minutes, playing basketball for 15 to 20 minutes, or running 1.5 miles in 15 minutes. These examples illustrate the balance between duration and intensity, with less strenuous activities requiring a longer duration to achieve the same caloric expenditure. Moderate amounts of activity will improve health for virtually everyone. Those who currently achieve moderate amounts of physical activity on a regular basis can obtain further benefit by increasing the duration, frequency, and intensity.

It is important to remember that it is not what we do on weekends or now and again that shapes our physical destiny, but that which we do virtually every single day of our lives.

Therefore, the journey to a transformed body begins where you stand right now. But taking that first step isn't always easy because it involves a life long commitment. However, once you begin, the perceived sacrifice will soon turn into a welcomed pleasure as you begin to feel better than you have perhaps in years.

It seems that we have plenty of reasons not to get started, nevertheless, let's examine a few of them more closely:

Too old. I've heard this one from everyone from the age of 30 to 80! The truth is it's *never* too late to begin an exercise program. The type of physical activity you choose, the duration and intensity may be at issue, but age is *never* a reason not to exercise at all.

Too fat. I notice that people at my health club come in all shapes and sizes these days. When I began working out at local gyms in Arizona as a teenager in the 80s, everyone was young and had a perfect or near-perfect body. But those days are over! Now, you're hard pressed to find a perfect body at the gym! There is something everyone can do to get fitter regardless of your size and level of fitness—whether it's walking in your neighborhood, going 2.5 miles on the treadmill, lifting 5-pound free weights, or doing mild water aerobics.

The rate of depression in the United States has increased more than 20-fold since 1950.

Too weak. Almost as instantly as you begin to exercise, this excuse will fade. Regular physical activity will result in greater strength and energy.

Too busy. Oddly enough, I *always* seem to find time to do the things that I really want to do. You have to ask yourself if 30 to 60 minutes a day is going to interfere with your life in a major way. What do you devote half and hour to an hour daily that offers you a greater reward than exercise?

Too tired. Most people are too tired *because* they don't exercise! Exercise will give you more energy and greater mental alertness. Toning your muscles and conditioning your heart, lungs and blood vessels will better equip you to deal with responsibilities and stress of daily living.

Begin by setting your exercise goals. This will help shape your exercise plan. Ask yourself why you need to exercise daily:
To feel better?
To look better?
To lose weight?
To have greater mobility?
To have more endurance?
To get stronger?
To have more energy?
To concentrate on your work better?
To reduce stress?
To elevate your mood?
To sleep better?
To ward off disease?
To live longer?

Perhaps your reasons are all of the above as they generally should be. Before you begin, you may want to check with your doctor for any physical limitations you may need to consider. You may also look into a local gym, join forces with a friend, get the whole family involved and consider the services of a personal trainer—at least to get you on the right track initially. But don't for a moment think that you need to belong to a fancy health facility or hire a costly personal trainer. Most of them got their certification in a weekend.

Let's begin by avoiding the "all or nothing" mentality and concentrate on internal motivators (like how energized exercise makes you feel). Tell people close to you about your new exercise plan and ask for their support. View exercise as a natural and necessary part of your life like eating, sleeping and working. Not only will exercise become a pleasurable habit in a matter of weeks; your very own body transformation will be well on its way!

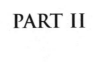

PART II

CHAPTER 7
DIGESTION TRANSFORMATION

One of the greatest energy sappers I know of is that awful fatigue and bloated feeling that accompanies poor digestion, which is usually due to poor food choices. Just imagine how you feel after a serious Thanksgiving dinner. You just want to collapse! And most of us do.

Indeed, it is important to recognize that at the root of your ability to thrive and survive in today's environment, is your digestive tract. It is your inner skin, the size of a tennis court! Your internal environment is created by your diet. It's that simple. If you put junk in, you create a junkyard. If you don't digest your food properly, toxins accumulate in the intestine and can be absorbed into the blood, leading to impaired immunity, disease, and premature aging. This is a high price to pay for perceived convenience, taste preference, and misguided eating habits.

You want to enable your body to more completely digest and absorb food in order to heal and regenerate itself. For this, we need to choose foods that boost digestion. You may even choose to take digestive enzymes. Such naturally derived enzymes decrease the allergy potential for foods eaten, thereby minimizing the potential irritation that characterizes conditions like ulcerative colitis, spastic colon, and irritable bowel syndrome.

Fresh raw foods contain natural enzymes that aid the body in digestion. These are not present in cooked and processed foods, which place an extra burden on the digestive system and set the stage for any of the degenerative diseases, like arthritis.

Plant enzymes help the body recover its own natural digestive abilities because they predigest food, taking a significant load off the stomach and small intestine. Enzymes have been used for centuries in many fermented food products such as soy sauce, miso, and cheese. Their use in these foods makes them more nutritious and easier to digest. Through modern technology, these enzymes have been concentrated in capsules and can now help support your better health at each meal. They are superior in most cases to enzymes such as porcine pancreatic enzymes, because they work in a much broader digestive pH range.

Plant digestive enzymes (2-5 caps; up to 20/day about 15-30 minutes before meals) will complete digestion of full spectrum foods, enhance assimilation, increase energy, and decrease exposure to allergens. Consuming raw foods (15-35 percent of your diet; more in summer, less in winter) will improve digestion and elimination,

> **A good diet is virtually valueless unless it can accomplish its purpose with proper digestion and absorption.**

provide live enzymes to support your vital force, provide greater nutrients, and will permit for less exposure to carcinogens.

At the beginning of each day, acidophilus is recommended —the friendly bacteria. You may choose to begin with a half-teaspoon upon rising and even half an hour to an hour before each meal. You may increase up to two teaspoons 2-3 times a day. This friendly microflora helps make antibodies, helps make vitamins, helps control unwanted bacteria, fungus and yeast, and will help neutralize some carcinogens and toxins.

Intestinal hygiene should be the buzz word of our age as so few people possess it and so many suffer crippling consequences due to a lack of it. To be healthy, the intestinal tract must be in proper working order *first.*

A good diet is virtually valueless unless it can accomplish its purpose with proper digestion and absorption. Food allergies are rampant among so many of us and causing us to be increasingly deprived of nutritious foods as a result. *A faulty digestive system contributes to deficiencies of vitamins, minerals and other vital nutrients which leads to numerous ailments and eventually, serious disease.*

Halitosis, or bad breath, is virtually always a consequence of putrefactive bacteria that is living on undigested food which forms foul smelling gasses that are released in exhaled air. A coated tongue is the result of bacteria growth of putrefactive bacteria in the intestine.

Our intestinal environment—specifically, the gastrointestinal tract, is an alimentary tube that extends from the lips to the anus. This area is filled with a mixture of foods, digestive ferments, liquids and solid waste. In other words, *if the digestive forces malfunction, you become a walking cesspool.* Problems arise when the delicate workings of the gastrointestinal tract are not working properly. They include indigestion, bloating, constipation, diarrhea, pancreatic disease, gallbladder disease, irritable bowel syndrome, infections, colitis, inflammatory bowel disorders, diverticulosis, and hemorrhoids, to name a few. Eventually, you can even develop candida, toxemia, or cancer.

The first stress is felt by the detoxifying organs, mainly the liver and kidneys. If these organs fail to detoxify and purify the blood stream, then the skin, glands and other eliminative organs are brought into jeopardy. At times, even the lungs in their endless process of purifying the blood through inhaling oxygen and exhaling carbon dioxide, help in ridding the body of gaseous toxins originated in the colon and small intestine.

This maldigestion/malabsorption problem is generally the result of a bad diet, antibiotic use, use of contraceptive pills and corticosteroids, lack of exercise, overeating, and consistently eating the same foods.

Fortunately, for every force there exists an equal and opposite force. In the GI tract, there is naturally about three-and-a-half pounds, or 11 billion constantly residing bacteria. Problems arise when friendly bacteria is not in sufficient supply to do the necessary job of effective digestion, absorption, and elimination. Billions of minute organisms form the friendly bacteria, which reside in the colon and under favorable conditions, multiply very rapidly. These microorganisms, which colonize and reproduce throughout your entire life, are called the *intestinal flora*.

The daily intake of foods which help promote the growth of these friendly bacteria are mandatory. They are primarily plain yogurt (always organic and preferably goat's milk), whey, buttermilk, acidophilus milk, kefir, and organic milk. However, if intestinal flora is quite low, then a supplementation with Lactobacillus acidophilus is vital. Be sure to use the freeze-dried variety found in powder form in dark glass bottles in the refrigerated section of better health food stores. Also be certain to check the expiration date as they do have a limited shelf life. Mix a full teaspoon in room-temperature water *only* and drink on an empty stomach, half an hour to an hour before meals. Guaranteed high potency supplements L. acidophilus, B. bifidium, and L. bulgaricus have been found effective in restoring the body's natural friendly flora balance. Please note that L. bulgaricus, unlike L. acidophilus, should be taken with meals or can be mixed with milk or fresh juices.

Friendly bacteria possesses vital therapeutic properties significantly affecting digestion, absorption, microbial infection, and immune system function, among other benefits and should be taken daily to help achieve optimal health.

In addition, I assure you, that no body transformation will take place without the vital role of *water*. We all know we need to drink it by now, but amazingly enough, we still *don't*. Water, second only to air, is the most important nutrient your body needs to survive. Yet, most of us aren't getting nearly enough of it. A lack of water not only causes dehydration, but an array of other illnesses and even death—much more so than a deficiency of any other nutrient. Consider the following:

- The average adult's body weight is 55-75 percent water (or about 10-12 gallons.)
- Average daily water loss is three quarts.
- Water regulates body temperature.
- Drinking plenty of water is the best skin moisturizer.
- Water carries nutrients and oxygen to cells.
- Fluid in blood transports glucose to working muscles.

- Water removes bodily wastes.
- A lack of water may make you feel very fatigued.
- A lack of water makes you feel bloated.
- Aging affects your body's water balance. With aging comes decreased thirst and urinary incontinence. Either or both has been shown to reduce the body's water content.
- The average person requires 8-12 eight-oz. glasses of water daily.
- The average person today drinks more soft drinks and alcohol than water.

Many will say: but all beverages contain water! This can pose a problem. Most beverages contain calories that are digested as food. The calories produce fat storage, blood sugar level disturbances, and decreased digestion. Pure water, however, travels right through the stomach with or without the presence of food. No processing or digesting is needed and it doesn't irritate or disturb body functions. On the other hand, sweetened drinks need extra water for metabolism. These and other beverages are further acid-forming in the stomach.

Sugar aside, diet sodas can be worse. Chemicals in drinks are added for flavor, color, preservation, and so forth,

Water, second only to air, is the most important nutrient your body needs to survive.

which generally irritate delicate stomach linings. Further, an extra burden is placed upon the liver and the kidneys as they must detoxify and eliminate the poisons.

How do you know if you are drinking enough water? One of the best indicators is your urine color. If your urine is a clear color and virtually odorless and you eliminate large quantities of it, this indicates a proper water balance. However, if you take vitamins, particularly B-vitamins and C, the urine will be dark as a result. In this case, frequency and quantity of elimination are the indicators. Also, if you are often fatigued, irritable and/or suffer many headaches, a chronic lack of water may definitely be a leading cause of it.

An avalanche of legislation recently passed through Congress in hopes that the Environmental Protection Agency (EPA) will set limits for drinking-water poisoning, especially for endocrine disrupting chemicals—chemicals that mimic human estrogen, frequently with hazardous results. These estrogen mimics are a very large group of chemicals that are known to disturb basic life functions by mimicking or blocking hormones. This can cause infertility and various reproductive problems, interfere with developing fetuses, increase the chance of hormone-related cancers and suppress the immune system.

Byproducts of industry and key ingredients in every day consumer products like plastics, lawn care chemicals and synthetic fertilizers have sufficiently poisoned our water supply. Additionally, millions of us drink tap water containing the protozoan parasite Cryptosporidium—a cause of serious illness and even death. This microscopic parasite had in 1995, for instance, harmed 45 million Americans. In Milwaukee alone, nearly half a million people fell ill and more than 100 died in 1993. Many other pathogens cause widespread public health problems. But you don't have to count yourself among the victims if you will only stop drinking tap water and drink primarily spring water instead.

Consider these options:

ARTESIAN WATER: derived from a well that taps a confined aquifer in which the water level stands above the top of the aquifer.

MINERAL WATER: derived from a geologically and physically protected underground water source. No minerals are added, but the water must contain a specific level of natural minerals and trace elements as found at the source.

SPARKLING WATER: contains naturally occurring carbon dioxide from the same source as the water.

SPRING WATER: flows naturally from an underground source to earth's surface. Water is bottled directly at the spring.

WELL WATER: collected from an aquifer from a hole constructed in the ground.

PURIFIED WATER: produced by distillation, reverse osmosis or other approved process. May be labeled as "distilled water" if it also has been boiled, vaporized, and condensed. Purified water is much preferred over tap water, but is essentially dead water, containing none of the life sustaining elements found in spring water.

If you are often fatigued, irritable and/or suffer many headaches, a chronic lack of water may be a leading cause of it.

A suggested meal plan to improve your digestion:

On rising:

Drink a glass of spring water at room temperature with one tea-spoon of acidophilus. Wait 30-60 minutes and drink a glass of diluted aloe vera juice and have breakfast.

Breakfast:

Fresh fruit in season of low glycemic index like berries or apples, and plain goat's milk yogurt* mixed with flax oil. Cup of green tea (you may sweeten with Stevia).

Supplements: vitamin-C,** vitamin-E, vitamin B-complex, a mul-tivitamin and mineral formula, Kyolic garlic capsule, after your meal.

Mid-morning:

A whole grain food. This may include a yeast-free multigrain toast, slow-cooked oatmeal, or a cup of brown rice with a bit of pure organic butter.

Supplements: apple pectin.

Lunch:

A leafy green salad with fresh lemon, extra virgin olive oil, fresh garlic and your favorite herbs and spices for dressing. (Avoid all commercially prepared salad dressings.) Also, choose fish or seafood such as tuna, salmon, cod, sea bass, or halibut. Cup of mint tea.

---

* *Goat's milk is alkaline and much easier to digest than cow's milk. Goat's milk products are also free of antibiotics and hormones so common in regular non-organic dairy products.*
** *Choose vitamin-C in calcium ascorbate form instead of ascorbic acid because it is not acid-forming in the stomach. Take all vitamins in solution, liquid or powder form for better absorption. Autopsies have been known to show hundreds on undigested hard vita-min pills in bodies.*

Supplements: digestive enzymes (before you eat), vitamin-C, vitamin-E, vitamin B-complex and Bio-bifidious (friendly bacteria) after your meal.

Mid-afternoon:
Crunchy raw vegetables with kefir*** cheese or plain yogurt. Cup of green tea or alfalfa tea.

Dinner:
A fresh vegetable salad sprinkled with nuts and seeds. Also have fish or beans or a whole grain food with the salad.
Supplements: digestive enzymes before you eat and vitamin-C, vitamin B-complex, a multivitamin and mineral, and Kyolic garlic after your meal.

Bedtime:
Drink a big glass of water with psyllium husks (natural fiber). If elimination is not complete, take a cup of senna tea (a natural laxative).

As you begin to transform your eating habits, always be mindful of the following:
Chew food very thoroughly.
Cut down on consumption of animal products.
Avoid refined sugars and all artificial sweeteners.
Avoid saturated oils and fats.
Limit salt.
Avoid soda, black tea, coffee, and alcohol.

*** *Kefir is a cultured food made by adding kefir grains (naturally formed milk proteins) to milk and letting the mix incubate overnight at room temperature to milkshake consistency. Kefir has 350mg of calcium per cup.*

Avoid fermented (bottled) fruit juices.

Drink 8-12 glasses of spring/mineral water daily.

Steam or grill your vegetables.

Eat whole grains only.

Eat organic poultry and meat.

Eat fruit by itself.

Eat extra virgin olive oil, pure organic butter, and limited nut oils (never peanut oil, margarine or fat substitutes).

Eat foods grown in your region whenever possible, and in its natural season.

Breathe deeply.

Exercise daily.

CHAPTER 8
IMMUNE FUNCTION TRANSFORMATION

T here was a time when I caught every cold that came along, had frequent sinus infections, and suffered an energy crisis that made the 1970s gasoline shortage seem pale by comparison. I sought help but every doctor dismissed it as "some bug that's going around." Often they would ask the infamous question, "Are you under stress, dear?" Frustrated, I fired back, "Doctor, are *you* under stress?" The only way to be completely free of stress is to be dead. We're all under stress but we shouldn't be under the kind of stress that debilitates.

I just didn't understand how I could have gone from force to fatigue so rapidly. For a long time, I feared the worst. At the time, my 42-year-old godmother suffered from fatigue and a general lack of well being for several years. She was patronized by the doctors to the extent of being sent to a psychiatrist. But it was all a prelude to lymph node cancer that resulted in 18 months of chemotherapy. She miraculously survived the cancer but lost her health and vitality forever.

Feeling abandoned by the medical experts, I began my own search for answers and was quite surprised to discover that there are so many potential opportunities for an immune breakdown throughout the body, which could cause a body transformation of an entirely undesirable kind, especially in the case of your digestive tract.

When your digestive system is weakened, you can contribute to the development of nutritional deficiencies, increase the amount of toxins you absorb, and decrease your overall immune function. You can also develop food allergies and autoimmune problems.

If properly cared for, your immune system can get smarter from experience— it can get better at identifying foreign substances, because some of your immune cells have memories for a lifetime. However, if they are bombarded with antigens and toxic substances, these immune cells can become hypersensitive, weakened or depleted, and unable to protect you properly.

Many digestive problems go undiagnosed in otherwise healthy people because they are so common—diarrhea, constipation, gas, cramping, indigestion, and fatigue. You can do plenty to support and correct your digestive immunity.

Although specific prescriptions are recommended for individual cases, plant digestive enzymes are frequently recommended to help take a significant burden off your digestive system. When you use enzymes, your body spends less energy on

> When your digestive system is weakened, you can contribute to the development of nutritional deficiencies, increase the amount of toxins you absorb, and decrease your overall immune function.

digestion, leaving more energy available for your immune system to make repairs, restore normal functions, or perform other life-enhancing tasks.

An all-purpose plant enzyme formula can help you digest all types of food better, but if you tend to eat lots of dairy products or beans that causes you embarrassment, or you find fats troublesome to digest, you can get specific enzyme combinations for your individual needs. These enzymes help you digest your favorite foods, providing you with greater nutrient and absorption potential while decreasing your exposure to allergic food particles.

It is vital to replenish your intestinal microflora, as discussed in the previous chapter. Did you know that when you are healthy, you have more beneficial bacteria in your digestive tract than you have cells in your body? They actually grow in your intestinal garden and they are essential for your life and well being.

You will benefit in many ways when you restore these bacteria to balance. They assist your digestion and absorption, immune function and modulation as well as vitamin and antibody production. They also prevent disease-causing bacteria from colonizing at your expense. They neutralize cancer-causing substances in your intestines.

I suggest that you take an intestinal microflora product, which contains FOS (fructooligosaccharides). FOS stimulates the growth of bifidobacterium (a beneficial microflora). Another way you can strengthen your digestion is by increasing the amount of fiber in your diet. You may want to do this gradually to avoid discomfort—and drink plenty of water because fiber absorbs many times its weight in water.

As you strengthen your immune system, you increase your ability to fight everything from yeast infections to cancer. Of course, you can improve your immunity with good nutrition. What you eat is the cornerstone of your immunity. The problem is that our diets have turned upside down. When food should be keeping us healthy, it's tragically making us sick. Our bodies hardly know what to do with our diet of refined food and fake food, so the bad things we eat clog up our system and contribute to all sorts of problems. We end up getting weaker and sicker and never understand why.

Dozens of natural foods help build up your immune system. The more of them you eat, the greater the chance for supercharged immunity. On the other hand, refined foods mostly tear down your immunity and make you weaker.

We must eat more whole foods that nature has given us and ideally, eat them when nature offers them—seasonally. Let vegetables and whole grains dominate your diet. After that comes beans (and other legumes), fruits, tubers, seeds and nuts, some fermented foods like plain yogurt, and kefir, and eggs. Meat and selected dairy products should bring up the rear. If they

Whenever you can, eat natural organic fruits, vegetables, dairy, poultry, and meat. They are free of pesticides, chemicals, hormones, steroids, and antibiotics.

are a part of your diet, enjoy, but buy organic and eat them sparingly and always with enzymes and added fresh vegetables.

A common phenomenon associated with a weakened immune system, especially as you get older, is the loss of the hormone called DHEA (dehydroepiandrosterone). DHEA is deficient in people as they age and is in some ways seen as an indication of your overall health. DHEA is a steroid hormone produced by your adrenal glands and it's the most abundant steroid in the human bloodstream. As you age, your DHEA levels fall quite considerably. Research has suggested that it may have significant anti-obesity, anti-cancer, anti-aging effects.

Immune-enhancing foods that you will want to make an important part of your diet include foods that contain high amounts of bioflavanoids, which have powerful antioxidant effects. More than 200 laboratory studies link diets rich in fruits and vegetables with a lower risk of cancer and immune dysfunction.

Different bioflavanoids from different foods and herbs often act on specific organs and tissues in your body. Bioflavanoids have an antibacterial effect and enhance the action of vitamin-C in your body. They are unique, in that their antioxidant capabilities have an exceptionally wide range—far wider than many other compounds like vitamin-E or selenium. Because your body can't produce them, you need to have them in your diet.

Foods with high bioflavanoid content are cabbage (with hearts), whole green peppers and citrus (including inner white membranes), parsley, carrots, broccoli, Brussels sprouts, turnips, parsnips, horseradish, scallions, onions, garlic, potatoes, yams, squash, pumpkin, soy sauce, eggplant, turmeric, sea vegetables, green tea, lemon juice, grapefruits, apples, and pears (with skin).

Whenever you can, eat natural organic fruits, vegetables, dairy, poultry, and meat. They are free of pesticides, chemicals, hormones, steroids, and antibiotics. Did you know that more than half of the antibiotic production in the United States is used in livestock feed? We know by now that indiscriminate use of antibiotics in humans impairs your immunity and breeds killer bugs. An excess of estrogen is implicated in several types of cancer, weight gain in women, and feminization of men. Organic foods contain more nutrients—around 200 percent more. If you have tasted them, you know there's no comparison.

Find out where there are local organic farmers' markets in your area. Support local farmers by calling your county agricultural extension agent (who should be able to direct you to local organic farmers) in addition to checking community health food and whole food stores. Also talk to your local grocery store management and ask that they carry organic products. I find that whenever I go to a regular grocery store (rarely for food, I might add), I dash through produce and dairy and tell anyone working there that I'm looking for organic versions of their available foods. I repeat myself at the checkout counter. When a clerk asks you if you found everything you wanted, tell him or her, "No. I want organic produce, milk and chicken." Let them all get familiar with the *word* organic, at least.

Your biggest internal exposure to harmful chemicals comes from your food. Animal products are responsible for roughly 75 percent of those in the average diet. By switching to organic food and eating moderate amounts of animal products, you can decrease your exposure to synthetic hormones, pesticides, and other harmful drugs by 75 percent.

You may have a good diet, but today most commercially grown food lacks essential nutrients. If the nutrition is not in the soil, it is not in the plant. Plants feed you directly, and indirectly when you consume the animals that eat them. Your health ultimately starts with soil health. When you think about it, soil, water and air feed *everything* on this planet.

If you count up pesticides, growth hormones, and additives in our food supply, we get too much of what we don't want as well. Your immune system, like a sports team, cannot play at its full potential if the starting players are missing. Even if the star players are ready, the team cannot live up to its potential without equipment and referees (supporting nutrients trace elements).

You can help prevent immune problems and fortify and build immune reserves by eating organic food and taking nutritional supplements. Start supplementing now and help reverse and correct health problems. It's never too late. It is part of the best health insurance plan you can have.

One of my favorite immune boosters is bee propolis. Bee propolis has a toning effect on the body. When propolis is taken regularly, it creates an antibiotic disease-fighting reaction to virtually any illness. Propolis has been proven to be effective against bacteria, viruses, and fungi because it activates the thymus gland and thus the immune system. The thymus gland consists primarily of developing lymphocytes, the white blood cells necessary for providing immunity against illness and infection.

Bee propolis, in thousands of documented cases and more than 500 published studies in medical journals all around the world, has proven itself not only a natural antibiotic, antiviral, anti-fungal source, but also as a potent cleanser of the body's cells and bloodstream. Further, it combats gastrointestinal disorders and clears troubled skin. Bee propolis, while effective for cell-blood cleansing and revitalizing simultaneously sweeps up harmful bacteria. Basically, propolis initiates an accelerated intracellular digestion of poison-forming substances, which allows this cleansing of cells and bloodstream.

Stomach ailments respond well to bee propolis as it provides a barrier to ulcer formation and speeds up recovery from an ulcer, should one be present. Gastrointestinal disorders relieved by bee propolis include nausea, heartburn, diminished appetite, and the balancing of the acid-alkaline state. In one particular study, after just 3-5 days on 20 drops of bee propolis taken three times a day, all subjects were completely free of pain and acidity was normalized while nausea and heartburn totally vanished. Researchers noted that, "Bee propolis is a medical preparation with bactericidal, anti-toxic, anti-inflammatory, and anesthetizing properties. In addition, it normalizes the secreting functions of the stomach. It can be recommended for the treatment of patients who are suffering from (all forms of) ulcers. Recovery occurs more quickly with treatment by propolis than it does with the use of common medicines."

What exactly is bee propolis? Specifically, it is resinous material that is gathered by bees from leaf buds and tree barks, mostly poplars. Propolis stems from the sap secreted by trees, which fights infections and disease, and it heals wounds. It is chestnut or greenish-brown in color and has a pleasant aroma of poplar buds, vanilla, and honey. Bee propolis has existed for more than 45 million years but has newly been scientifically documented for its healing ability.

To bees, propolis is a natural cement for their hives that protects them from invaders and concomitants, thus making the beehive the most sterile environment in the animal kingdom. In people, the bioflavanoids in propolis are virtually identical to the action of aspirin in that they block the same enzyme that controls pain and fever.

Bee propolis may be taken in various forms. These include lozenges for sore throats, coughs, and colds, capsules or tables for convenience, tincture which can be diluted and used as a gargle, salve for soothing the skin, granules for chewing, and, powder that can be mixed with water or fresh juice for easy digestion. Regardless of form, bee propolis can certainly transform your body for the better without absolutely any documented side effects. You can start supplementing now and help protect your health for the future. Prevention is the key to a prosperous longevity.

The following supplementation is recommended for a stronger immune system. This basic yet comprehensive program will not expose you to too much of the fat-soluble vitamins that can be harmful if stored in the body.

Green superfoods: These are one of nature's most nutrient-rich foods. All green foods contain high amounts of chlorophyll. Chlorophyll is almost identical in molecular structure and chemical content to hemoglobin, the basic building block in all human and animal red blood cells. In fact, chlorophyll is often called the *blood* of plants.

Though chlorophyll is not technically a vitamin, its importance to your optimal nutrition is now widely accepted. The benefits of chlorophyll include its ability to remove toxic pesticide and drug residues from your system, as well as to bind with radioactive materials and remove them from your body. Chlorophyll is one of the best internal cleansing products available, making it even more important that you take it in today's unnatural world. It is known for its powerful detoxifying and important anti-cancer properties without sideeffects.

We are urged to eat at least five fresh fruits and vegetables each day. Fortunately, you can compensate for not always being able to make the BIG FIVE every day by taking your choice of these green superfoods: chlorella and spirulina, barley grass, wheat grass, blue-green algae, and alfalfa.

Take these green superfoods in the morning and again at lunch or in the mid-afternoon. They can stabilize your energy level, help detoxify your system, and add energy-important nutrients, trace elements, and phytochemicals.

Phycocyanin, found in some large algae, helps maintain your normal white blood cell count. Spirulina has 60 percent complete digestible protein, more than any other food on the planet.

I believe that the "green gold of the future" is the superfood blue-green algae called spirulina. This single-cell organism, in fact, the lowest thing on the food chain, contains a complete protein that is richer than steak, abundant in organically complex minerals, a vast array of essential vitamins and crucial enzymes. By all means an ideal food, spirulina is important for maintaining your target weight, controlling

You may have a good diet, but today most commercially grown food lacks essential nutrients.

allergies, correcting visual disturbances, carbohydrate disorders, anemia, and many other forms of disease.

Spirulina comes from warm, alkaline, fresh waters. It is billed as the food of the future due to its incredible ability to synthesize high-quality concentrated food more effectively than any other algae. Spirulina is 65-71 percent "complete" protein (compared to beef's 22 percent) and contains all the essential amino acids in perfect balance.

Spirulina's photosynthetic conversion rate is 8-10 percent compared to a mere 3 percent of land growing plants. Further, it is a source of vitamin B12, a nutrient we consume primarily through red meat. A teaspoon of spirulina contains nearly three times the U.S. Recommended Daily Allowance of this vitamin and has more than twice the amount of B12 found in the same protein of liver.

High concentrations of amino acids, chelated minerals, pigmentations, complex natural plant sugars, trace elements, and enzymes are provided by spirulina in an easily assimilated form.

The Japanese medical establishment has shown a great interest in spirulina and has reported on its numerous great effects in top medical journals. They include:

Diabetes: the easily assimilated sugars of spirulina helped maintain the blood glucose levels steady. The algae helped stop food cravings, which resulted in weight loss and a reduced need for insulin.
Anemia: the chlorophyll, vitamin B12, folic acid, and protein content of spirulina was able to increase red blood cell volume and oxygen carrying capacity within a month.
Liver disease: the liver is dependent upon high quality and easy-to-digest protein and concentrated vitamins when toxins and

infections are assaulting it. The nutritional content of spirulina boosts the liver's recuperative powers.

Ulcers: two grams of spirulina were able to cure all symptoms of gastric ulcers. In addition, seven out of nine cases of duodenal ulceration were completely cured in a reported study. Spirulina's chlorophyll helps coat the irritated stomach lining, inhibits mal-adoptive pepsin secretions and is an ulceration inhibitor.

Pancreatitis: the pancreas is the organ entrusted with blood sugar regulation and synthesis of many digestive enzymes. Dietary abuses, especially over-consumption of sugar and alcohol, can exhaust the pancreas and cause it to self-destruct. Spirulina can forestall pancreatic exhaustion and return balance to the flow of enzymatic secretions.

Visual problems: 90 percent of geriatric cataracts were improved with a combination of medication and spirulina.

Leukocyte loss prevention: radiation and chemotherapy treatment for cancer often results in undesirable reduction of defensive white cells. But in studies, only 2-3 grams of spirulina had slowed this loss of white blood cells.

Heavy metal poisoning: The use of spirulina can stimulate the excretion of some contaminants, notably cadmium, at an acceler-ated rate. The algae have also successfully excreted lead and mer-cury in test patients.

Senility: most cases of senility are the result of prolonged and sub-tle nutritional deficiencies. Alzheimer's disease is related to aluminum poisoning. When a chronic shortage of nutrients is a contributing factor to mental deterioration, the concentrated proteins, vitamins, and minerals of spirulina can potentiate restoration of normal function. The presence of amino acids that helps regulate mood and supply the nerve nutrient inositol found in spirulina can help sharpen brain function.

Spirulina is not a magic solution but a high quality nutritional food and adjunct to conventional treatments. Therapeutic doses are usually 6-10 grams (12-20 tablets) daily, which is also the amount that athletes and "health nuts" take. However, since spirulina is a *food*, "dosages" have little value. Eight-20 tablets are adequate for most individuals.

I rotate spirulina, chlorella, and Green Energy foods every few months. When I want extra protection and energy, I use combinations of them at the same time. Take them often and take them regularly. This is real immune insurance.

Take a complete multi vitamin/mineral: For proper immune function, a daily multi-vitamin/mineral is not an option, it's a necessity. Take it in liquid or capsule form or powdered multi-vitamin/mineral—no horse pills!

Take antioxidants: Take with meals two or three times a day, as directed. Antioxidants neutralize free radicals. They act as scavengers, helping to prevent cell and tissue damage that could harm the cells and led to disease. Vitamin E is the most abundant fat-soluble antioxidant, and vitamin C is the most water-soluble antioxidant in the body. Others include bioflavanoids, folic acid, green tea, garlic, and selenium.

Even though you have some 100 trillion cells in your body, you really don't have any to spare. The greatest enemy to your cells is free radicals—unpaired electrons that speed up the process of biological aging and the wear and tear on our bodies. Free radicals search and attack virtually every molecule in your body, including fats, protein, and even the DNA within cells. Free radicals, in search of their missing electron, roam through our bodies and are often the culprits in cellular damage, which accounts for why antioxidants—nutrients that prevent or counteract free radical damage—are vital for cellular protection.

Co-enzyme Q10: This plays a vital role in immunity. People over the age of 50 or with impaired health often have low levels. Taking co-enzyme Q10 has been shown to improve immunity and speed up healing. Dosages are from 30-100mg daily. I suggest starting with 30mg twice a day.

Essential Fatty Acids (EFSs): These are the good fats that are our number-one dietary deficiency. These polyunsaturated fats are vital to body function. They decrease inflammation, help regulate your hormone levels, can decrease tumor growth and help your body make sense and use interferon, an anti-viral protein. EFA's include both Omega-6 (linoleic) and Omega-3 (alpha-linoleic) fatty acids. Together, they are used to create prostaglandins, the hormone-like chemical messengers responsible for regulating blood pressure, oxygen transport, pain, and inflammation. But EFAs main function is to maintain the liquid barrier surrounding each cell—the cell membrane, and to transport waste and

Chlorophyll is almost identical in molecular structure and chemical content to hemoglobin, the basic building block in all human and animal red blood cells.

nutrients, amino acids, hormones, minerals, vitamins, and water in and out of cells. Remember, *the lining of every cell in the body is made of fat.* Cells can communicate with each other when membranes are fluid. Polyunsaturated fats are fluid; saturated fats are solid. Low levels of EFAs adversely affect brain function and cardiovascular, inflammatory, and immune systems. Skin problems, depression, PMS, learning disabilities, and a host of additional ailments can be directly linked to a lack of *good fat* in our diets.

You will note throughout this dietary program that we are to use only fats from extra virgin olive oil, flax oil, and oils found naturally in fish, nuts, and avocados. These are the fats we really need. Too much of the wrong kind of fats and oils are being consumed today. Many contemporary diseases are generally diseases of fatty degeneration and essential fatty acid deficiencies. Our diets are overloaded with Omega-6 fatty acids, leaving us deprived of the Omega-3 fatty acids, which primarily come from flaxseed and its oil and from deep-water fish.

The Omega-3 and Omega-6 fatty acid families are constituents of the raw materials or precursors to prostaglandins, which are the very active biological substances that regulate nearly every body function, so are at least supportive in controlling the inflammatory process, the immune system, the neural circuits of the brain, the cardiovascular system (including cholesterol levels), the digestive and reproductive systems, and, the body thermostat and calorie loss mechanism.

A lack of EFAs in your diet can cause a reduction in number and size of brain cells as well as lack of communication between the brain cells that can involve problems in learning, growing, and thinking.

Essential fatty acids are those fatty acids essential to the body. But EFAs are not produced by the body and therefore need to be consumed. Flax seed and flax seed oil are an ideal source of Omega-3 fatty acids because of their two components, linoleic acid (LA) and alpha linoleic acid (LNA), are essential fatty acids. Flaxseed contains possibly the highest quality of LNA known in any natural product. Additionally, Omega-3 fatty acids can be found in seeds and plants from cold climates, green leafy vegetables, and oils extracted from cold water fish like mackerel, salmon, tuna, and cod.

Unfortunately, due to food processing, most of what we eat has been adulterated. To make matters worse, there is a concerned effort to remove all of the Omega-3 oil-containing foods since they spoil rapidly because the unsaturated fatty acids attract oxygen and become oxidized or turn rancid. However, it is precisely this feature of attracting oxygen easily that makes unsaturated fatty acids so vital to our well being, since they aid in oxygen delivery in the body.

Therefore, since EFAs form the membranes of every one of the billions of cells in our body, control the way cholesterol works in our system, make up a very large part of the brain's active tissues, and are the only fats that play a key role in regulating the cardiovascular, immune, digestive, and reproductive functions, inflammation and healing, functioning of the brain, controlling of body heat, and calorie burning, we should all ingest a tablespoon of flax seed oil daily as well as increase our consumption of cold water fish.

All of the above mentioned needs to be a part of your daily dietary routine to help build a strong immune system that will lead to body regeneration and thus transformation from within. This will go a long way towards helping you achieve high energy, vitality, and optimal health.

A suggested meal plan to help improve your immune function:

<u>On Rising:</u>
Drink a glass of spring water at room temperature with one
rounded teaspoon of acidophilus.

<u>Breakfast:</u>
Fresh fruit in season. A tablespoon of bee propolis and aloe vera*
juice.
Supplements: vitamin C**, vitamins B-complex, vitamin E, Co-
enzyme Q10, essential fatty acids, vitamin A, a multi vitamin-
mineral, kelp, Kyolic garlic.

<u>Mid-morning:</u>
Hot cup of potassium broth (made from simmered vegetables,
primarily root vegetables) and a glass of fresh carrot juice.
Echinacea and astragalus extract in a small amount of room temperature water. Green barley tablets.

<u>Lunch:</u>
Leafy green salad with extra virgin olive oil, flax oil, fresh lemon
juice, and garlic. (The redder the lettuce, the higher the nutrient content.) Also, choose a protein from a choice of fish,
seafood, chicken or tofu.*** Add steamed vegetables of your lik-
ing—always fresh, rarely frozen and never canned. Hot cup of

---

* *Aloe vera juice has long been in use for burns and skin care in gel form, but aloe juice
is excellent for its digestive and laxative properties.*
** *For a weakened immune system, you may gradually increase vitamin C intake from
5,000-20,000mg daily (always taken with food).*
*** *Tofu is made from soy beans, water, and nigari, a mineral-rich precipiate. Tofu is an
excellent meat replacement. Combined with whole grains, tofu yields a complete protein
without the fat or cholesterol but with all the calcium and iron while being low in calories.*

Pau de Arco**** tea.

Supplements: vitamin C, vitamin E, vitamin B-complex, zinc, copper, vitamin A, raw liver extract.

Many contemporary diseases are generally diseases of fatty degeneration and essential fatty acid deficiencies.

Mid-afternoon:

Spirulina and a whole grain food such as multigrain bread. Or, have raw nuts (but no peanuts). Also, have a cup of hot potassium broth or a freshly squeezed juice such as apple or carrot and ginger. Echinacea and ginkgo extract.

Dinner:

Bean and/or lentil soup cooked with hearty vegetables like potatoes, carrots, leeks, and cabbage. Or, have fish or seafood with a green salad and brown rice.

Supplements: vitamin C, a multi vitamin-mineral, manganese, Kyolic garlic, evening primrose oil,***** and ginkgo extract.

Bedtime:

Aloe vera juice and fresh squeezed pineapple or papaya juice with grape seed extract. Also a glass of room temperature water with a tablespoon of psyllium husk or a mild senna tea.

**** *Pao de Arco is an excellent blood purifier.*
***** *Evening primrose oil aids in weight loss and reduces high blood pressure. It is also a natural estrogen promoter that is helpful in treatment of hot flashes, menstrual problems, skin disorders, and many other disorders.*

CHAPTER 9
THE ACID-ALKALINE BALANCE

When we complain of an acid stomach to the doctor, we inevitably get a prescription for a powerful antacid drug. Sometimes, they are the same drugs used to treat ulcers and other digestive disorders. Most of us, however, can control this acidity with proper food choices. Many people also end up in emergency rooms thinking they are having heart problems (about 50 percent of the time) when what they are really suffering from is acid indigestion! I was among them—more than once. But how often has your doctor checked the acidity level in your urine, saliva, and blood? If you go to an allopathic doctor, which most people do, the answer is most likely, "never."

The body is programmed to keep a cell healthy within very narrow limits. Temperature, blood chemistry, and homeostasis determine healthy cells. Now, in western medicine, hardly anyone pays attention to pH. However, this is very important because it's one of the three parameters blood, urine, and saliva by definition. Therefore, pH would provide totally different information from blood, urine and saliva. Hence, to the best of my estimation, to measure pH, only a couple of hundred doctors across the United States rely on a bioelectronic machine that determines your body's pH level. Bioelectronic machines measure parameters of pH (acid-alkaline balance), redox potential (the amount of oxygen or lack of oxygen), and resistivity (the amount of mineralization or demineralization) of blood, urine, and saliva.

Fatigue or general exhaustion is the main reason most people go to see their doctor these days. One of the leading causes of fatigue is increased acidity of blood. If you are overworked, over stressed and overfed—primarily with acid-forming foods like meats, dairy and sugars, and fermented foods like bottled juices and pickled foods—you undoubtedly have acidity of the blood. This acid condition of the blood causes exhaustion first, and many health problems and even dangerous disease conditions later.

An acid condition inhibits nerve action and an alkaline condition stimulates nerve action. If you have an acid-alkaline balance, you can think and act well and possess optimal energy. But if you have an acidic condition, you simply cannot think clearly, act quickly or decisively. Quite possibly the number-one consequence of acidity is a depression of the central nervous system. Fatigue, depression, muscle stiffness, spasms, and headaches are all too common when you are acidic. Lower back pain—of which some 80 percent of the

> Many people end up in emergency rooms thinking they are having heart problems (about 50% of the time) when what they are really suffering from is acid indigestion!

American population suffers from at one time or another—neck and shoulder tension, osteoporosis, and a type of toxemia that is brought on because the kidneys are overtaxed by having to excrete the acids, all result from this acid-alkaline imbalance.

The over-acidic live with some stomach aches, nausea, vomiting, and chest pain. Gastritis and ulcers thrive in an acid environment. When the body adopts and then adapts to illness and degenerative disease, the urine will be very acidic and the blood will be very alkaline and oxidized (lack of oxygen). It has frequently been noted that one of the most important causes of cancer and other degenerative diseases is the cumulative effect of a disastrous acidic urine with an alkaline blood condition. By maintaining an acid-alkaline balance, wisdom has it that you can, to a large extent, prevent virtually any illness from the flu to cancer to heart disease.

Thus, in order for us to be healthy and operating optimally, our blood must be kept at a slightly alkaline level of pH 7.3; the urine should be slightly acidic at pH 6.8; and, saliva should be at pH 6.5. This is primarily achieved by breathing fresh air deeply, drinking proper amounts of pure water, eating a balanced and healthy diet, and exercising every day.

Although one must allow for *biological individuality*—after all, we are all different—the consensus is that our diets should consist of about 80 percent alkaline-producing foods, and 20 percent acid-forming foods. In reality, this is usually just the opposite. Watch television at virtually any given hour and note how many antacid products and painkillers are offered!

In addition to the acidic foods we eat, our bodies are continuously producing acid waste products of metabolism that has to be neutralized one way or another to sustain itself. As a result, we require a constant feeding of alkaline foods to neutralize this ongoing acid generation. Whether we live or die, thrive or merely limp along, is determined by our body's capability to maintain approximately an ideal 7.3 blood pH level.

Alkaline is the normal pH for all the tissues and fluids in the body, except the stomach. And there certainly is a lot of fluid—approximately 70 percent of our body weight in fact, the same percentage of water to land on Earth. However, most of us are acidic and this causes the blood to take alkaline-forming elements from the digestive enzyme system of the small intestine. This leads to trouble. The pancreatic and liver digestive enzymes, which depend on a proper alkaline pH of the small intestine, now doesn't possess an alkaline pH that's effective enough for it to function optimally. In a nutshell, this results in very poor digestion.

Therefore, a balanced blood pH is vital to proper digestion since otherwise important nutrients would not be assimilated and delivered to their desired places. Digestive disorders mean electrolyte imbalances—especially that of sodium, potassium, magnesium, and calcium ions. Such an electrolyte imbalance disturbs the fluid transport system in the body, which then results in nutrient malabsorption and

> If you have an acid-alkaline balance, you can think and act well and possess optimal energy.

poor waste elimination. When these alkaline reserves are low or depleted, the body becomes more acidic. The body then slowly depletes the calcium, magnesium, sodium, and potassium from the nerve cells to neutralize the blood.

This is when the nervous system begins to break down. Alertness suffers. Thinking becomes slow. Lethargy sets in. And, in severe cases, coma could occur below an acid blood pH of 6.95. Mental slowness and fogginess are common among those whose diet is too acidic.

Numerous diseases are the result of the body's attempt to rebalance its internal environment. There are many reasons why an acidic system is fertile ground for disease. The more acidic you become, the harder it is for your body to maintain a blood pH of 7.3. Degeneration starts at pH 7.8 for blood, pH 5.45 for urine, and pH 7.05 for saliva. For example, one way your body begins to compensate for pH imbalance is by depositing excess acid substances in the tissues and joints—eventually leading to arthritis, in this example.

Poor diet is the leading cause of an acid-alkaline imbalance. If your nourishment primarily consists of meats, fish, breads, pasta, dairy, convenience foods, processed foods, coffee, and sodas, and if you are taking synthetic vitamins or over-the-counter or prescription drugs, clearly you will become acidic, if you aren't already. On the other hand, those who eat mainly fresh fruits, vegetables, fresh juices, sea vegetables, and miso (primarily vegetarians) can become too alkaline.

Symptoms of excess alkalinity include an over excitability of the nervous system. A slightly elevated alkaline pH can produce a certain sense of euphoria. But in a graduated state of alkalinity, muscle twitching, muscle pain and spasm, anxiety, a spacey feeling, and even extreme nervousness can occur. As in acid conditions, there is an increase in colds and flu with excessive alkalinity.

Naturally, we are acid and alkaline simultaneously. The goal is to achieve the desired balance. Hence, the vital importance of the proper diet. When the blood pH is at 7.3, all the enzymes and electrolytes of the various digestive systems, organ systems, and glandular systems perform at peak level.

As a preventive or corrective measure, you can do a daily urine pH test. A kit may be obtained in most pharmacies. However, if you suspect an acid-alkaline imbalance, a doctor (preferably a good homeopath, naturopath, or Doctor of Oriental Medicine) can perform a blood pH test for best results and guided recovery.

Your acid-alkaline balance is something you should get checked regularly along with other vital signs. By middle age, you don't want to just wake up one day to discover that you have become diabetic, arthritic, acidic, or that your arteries are clogged. When you know where you stand, you know how to help yourself. There is no reason why anyone today should be ignorant about preventive medicine—when we become sick, it can be too late.

To be healthy, we can transform our body by thinking constructively, acting according to our own inner truths, and by taking responsibility for ourselves. The nice thing about self-responsibility is that we have a choice. We can choose to eat good food. We can choose to sleep. And, we can choose our attitude about any situation. We are responsible for the way we feel emotionally and how the physical body will support us.

To become more alkaline:

1. Eliminate or decrease the consumption of meat, chicken, and fish.
2. Eat less protein of any source.
3. Increase consumption of olive oil and flaxseed oil.
4. Decrease intake of all other fats.
5. Eliminate or decrease all pasteurized dairy.
6. Eliminate all sugar containing products.
7. May take raw honey.
8. Consume 5-10 servings of fresh organic raw fruits and vegetables daily.
9. Eat sprouted greens, alkaline-forming nuts, seeds, and grains.
10. Take alkalinizing juices and herbs such as fresh lemon juice, wheatgrass and cabbage juice, and chaparral tea.
11. Detox your kidneys, liver, and bowels.
12. Breathe deeply throughout the day; do deep breathing exercises upon rising in the morning.

To become more acidic:

1. Take 1 teaspoon of organic apple cider vinegar in a glass of water five minutes before meals.
2. Increase protein consumption.
3. Drink yellow dock tea or take herbal drops.
4. Consume cranberry juice, onions, and garlic.
5. Take vitamin A.

Very alkaline-forming foods:

Figs, chaparral tea, carrot juice, beet juice, cabbage juice, vegetable juices, miso, vitamin K, calcium ascorbate form of vitamin C, ginger, and wheatgrass juice.

Alkaline-forming foods:
Cherries, ripe fruit, bananas, strawberries, most vegetables, tomatoes, cabbage, millet, buckwheat, raw dairy, bean sprouts, string beans, soy beans, lima beans, spinach, chestnuts, sprouted almonds, Brazil nuts, egg whites, alfalfa sprouts, sunflower sprouts, honey, tofu, herb teas.

Very acid-forming foods:
Unripe cranberries, watermelon seed, yellow dock herb, walnuts, peanuts, apple cider vinegar, sauerkraut, fermented foods, egg yolk, vitamin A, meat, chicken, and fish.

Acid-forming foods:
Unripe fruit, prunes, plums, yeast, pasteurized dairy, animal fat, most beans, lentils, kidney beans, soy sauce, soft drinks, prescription drugs, alcohol, peas, most cooked grains, asparagus, most nuts, most seeds.

Quite possibly the number-one consequence of acidity is a depression of the central nervous system.

A suggested meal plan to regulate your acid-alkaline balance:

For the <u>FIRST DAY ONLY</u>: A 24-hour liquid fast to help eliminate acid wastes.

<u>On rising:</u>

Drink a glass of spring water with the juice of two fresh lemons and a teaspoon of blackstrap molasses.*

Supplements: vitamin C, vitamin E, a multi vitamin-mineral.

<u>Mid-morning:</u>

In the blender: 1 papaya, 1 pineapple, 1 large orange, slice of fresh ginger. Or, 1 bunch of grapes, 3 apples, 1 pint of strawberries, and 4 sprigs of fresh mint. Also, alfalfa ** tablets.

<u>Lunch:</u>

Freshly juiced apple, pineapple, papaya or cucumber.

Barley green*** tablets.

<u>Mid-afternoon:</u>

Ginger**** tea.

---

* Blackstrap molasses (unsulphured) is rich in minerals and vitamins. Molasses has more calcium than milk, more iron than eggs, and more potassium than any other food. It contains all the B-complex vitamins and vitamin E.

** Alfalfa is one of the world's richest mineral foods, pulling up earth sources from root depths as great as 130 feet. It is the basis for liquid chlorophyll, with a balance of chemical and mineral constituents almost identical to human hemoglobin. Alfalfa is excellent for a wide range of skin and intestinal disorders, arthritis, liver problems, breath, and body odor.

*** Barley green contains a broad spectrum of concentrated vitamins, minerals, enzymes, proteins, and chlorophyllins. It has 11 times the calcium of cow's milk, five times the iron of spinach, and seven times the vitamin C and bioflavanoids as orange juice. Latest research shows that barley green can help repair damaged DNA and it also helps slow down the aging process. Barley green is an ideal food source and anti-inflammatory agent for healing stomach and duodenal ulcers, hemorrhoids, and for pancreas infections.

**** Ginger possesses therapeutic properties for digestion, hypertension, and headaches. Ginger is a warming circulator stimulant and body cleansing herb.

Dinner:

Fresh squeezed papaya and pineapple juice. Also, spirulina tablets.

Bedtime:

Mint tea.

In addition: Drink 8-10 full glasses of water throughout the day.

The following day, after your cleanse:

On rising:

Drink a glass of spring water with a rounded teaspoon of acidophilus.

Breakfast:

Fresh fruit in season and plain yogurt.

Supplements: vitamin C, vitamin E, vitamin B-complex, and ginger tea.

Mid-morning:

Hot potassium broth, goat's milk and/or goat's milk yogurt. Or, kefir cheese on whole grain toast. Cup of elder flower tea.

Supplements: kelp and vitamin A.

Lunch:

Leafy green salad with flax oil, lemon, garlic, and seasonings of your choice. A lima bean salad with lightly steamed crunchy vegetables. Ginger tea.

Supplements: vitamins B-complex, a multi vitamin-mineral, potassium.

Mid-afternoon:

Fresh squeezed papaya or pineapple or apple juice. Spirulina tablets and a cup of fennel* tea.

Dinner:

Basmati** rice, your choice of vegetables from the "alkaline foods" list and egg whites. Chaparral tea or extract.

Supplements: vitamin C, vitamin E, vitamins B-complex, vitamin A, kelp, and a multi vitamin-mineral.

Bedtime:

Alfalfa tea.

---

* *Fennel can be used as an appetite suppressant. It promotes the functioning of the kidneys, liver, and spleen and also clears the lungs. Relieves abdominal pain, colon disorders, and gas. Useful for acid stomach.*
** *Basmati rice originated from India and is now grown as a hybrid in Texas. This is the Mercedes of rice—far superior and easier to digest than regular brown rice.*

CHAPTER 10
ENERGY TRANSFORMATION

Your well being rests squarely on your shoulders. Information and alternatives to standard medical care is available to virtually everyone today, all it takes is determination and time. In other words, how much time and attention is a healthy mind and body worth to you?

The well informed always rely on the natural first, like the healing powers of herbs and plants to help them better cope with the demands that modern living imposes on their health. Since lack of energy and general fatigue is our number-one complaint, the well informed tend to rely on the combinations of the extracts that were so effectively used in China some 1,000 years ago before the fall of Rome. Chinese practitioners manage to control the flow of energy in the body to cure disease, increase vitality, and longevity.

For this reason, herbalists and doctors of Oriental Medicine are in great demand among those whose vitality is essential to their success. They focus on the medicinal constituents of herbs and use them in assisting the body to function harmoniously.

Chinese medicine recognizes the body's vital energy, or life force, known as chi, which is a balance of hot and cold, moist and dry, yin and yang. Experts believe an imbalance of this vital energy causes the body to malfunction on various levels.

Therefore intervention with specific formulas derived from plants can restore balance. This results in disease prevention and health restoration. Whether you are stressed-out, exhausted, depressed and burned-out, or plagued by arthritis, chronic back pain, migraines, heart disease and in some cases, even cancer, these doctors can usually provide great health benefits. But most importantly, they can help you by seeing to it that you never encounter such ailments in the first place.

As we get older, years of poor diet and bodily abuses begin to manifest themselves in the form of chronic ills. Orthodox doctors, the alopaths that we all go to, are still among the best in the world when it comes to diagnosing our ailments, but the problem is that they can do little, if anything, to bring us back to optimal health. Generally, they treat symptoms of the problem, which only masks them and does not provide a long-term solution.

But consider what the ancient Chinese thought about such a system. Doctors would be retained to keep people healthy. They were held personally

> The major difference between Chinese medicine and Western medicine is that the Chinese specialize in health while the Western focuses on disease.

responsible and accountable when their patients became ill! A physician who discovered symptoms of disease was considered inferior for not having prevented it. This is plainly stated by the Yellow Emperor's chief medical advisor in his, *Internal Book of Hung Di:*

"To administer medicines to diseases which have already developed and to suppress revolts (symptoms) which have already developed is comparable to the behavior of those persons who begin to dig a well after they have become thirsty, and of those who begin to make their weapons after they have already engaged in battle. Would these actions not be too late?"

The major difference between Chinese medicine and Western medicine, is that the Chinese specialize in health while the Western focuses on disease. Doctors of Oriental medicine achieve health by supporting the body's natural order (enhancing immunity) and by minimizing the potential for disease. Observation is a key element of diagnosis. The tongue, eyes, skin color, hearing, pulse, age, weight, body type, voice, hair, posture, and body odor are among things analyzed. With great perception aimed at early detection, doctors of Oriental medicine have great success healing viruses, bacterial infections, and other external body invaders. Herbs are used not only to treat a specific ailment, but all parts of the body that may be affected. This restores overall balance and a well-balanced body can heal itself more efficiently.

Body transformation cannot take place without preventive medicine. This follows two primary principles: you must engage in a healthy personal lifestyle as described throughout this book, and your doctor must detect weaknesses in you before they turn into disease. You are responsible for a smart diet, adequate exercise, proper rest, deep breathing, a controlled sex life, and other regular preventive measures. A personal, daily approach to preventive care is mainly what will keep chronic and degenerative illness away. At the same time, you are generally healthier, more energized, alert, and effective in your daily life.

Your doctor must be skilled enough to recognize the subtle signs of pre-clinical symptoms. Unfortunately, most Western medical doctors do a battery of blood tests, x-rays and if they can't find anything there, usually tell the patient that there's nothing wrong with him. But, doctors of Oriental medicine look for any and all indicators that expose a vulnerability to future illness. Hence, if early warnings are corrected in time, you do not have to endure suffering and premature aging.

We are faced with premature aging, no matter what our age, as perhaps never before. It's not just a matter of weight gain, muscle loss, wrinkles, sagging skin, or graying hair. Far too often, we are faced with debilitating illness and early death. A shocking 90 percent of the Western population living in cities is in a pre-cancerous state. This is largely due to toxicity—a toxic environment, an adulterated food supply, lack of exercise, lack of sound sleep, and impure blood.

These things lead to poor digestion and an overall toxic body. If digestion is poor, the immune system is going to be bad. Is it any wonder then that one out of every three Americans today is diagnosed with a deadly disease? If you don't want to get cancer, you better make darn sure that your blood is clean. Astonishingly, according to experts across the board, 80 percent of cancer is entirely preventable if we would engage in the healthy lifestyle primarily described in this book.

How can we get closer to accurately identifying our true state of physical and mental health in order to increase our energy and vitality? Let's consider our own personal "biological terrain."

Biological terrain is a simple representation of the body's tendency towards the manifestation of a particular metabolic imbalance. Most simply stated, biological terrain is like the soil in which a farmer must grow his crops. If the soil is too acidic or too alkaline, or if there are not adequate minerals, a crop like corn or soybeans cannot grow. However, if it manages to develop, it will be very susceptible to specific invading insects or disease entities. On the other hand, if we can change the chemistry of the soil, we can scientifically alter the health and vitality of the crop. This exact concept, when related to the internal environment of the body, is in fact the definition of biological terrain.

Alongside the well-accepted diagnostic procedures of microbiology—the study of cells and the use of x-rays—there can be nothing more natural than the ability to understand health and disease through standardized measured parameters. In our current highly technical electronic society, the concept of numerically determining the state of physical well being is not a 21st century fantasy, but a reality today. With our present knowledge, doctors of Oriental medicine can accurately determine specific parameters, which reflect the body's state of wellness. Thus, a biological imbalance that can lead to illness can be precisely calculated by testing and utilizing the bodily fluids of saliva, blood, and urine. Information derived from these three bodily fluids can then be graphed in an easy-to-read and comprehensible format, thereby determining the prosperity for a particular disease state of biological imbalance. Once the doctor has graphed the patient's values he can then, within a very safe and accurate degree, predict the probability of the metabolic destination. In other words, it can be determined if your body is transforming in a positive or negative direction.

Analyzing the biological terrain does not and cannot diagnose any specific disease. Analyzing the terrain of the body gives us no more information about a particular disease state than the soil analysis tells us the *exact* insect that may be currently invading its leaves. Then, if understanding biological terrain does not give us the specifics we seek, why do we feel its value is on par with other medically proven systems of analysis?

Let's compare biological terrain data with the information received from a standard chemistry profile. This highly respected analytical tool is utilized each and every day by thousands of physicians around the world, but does it diagnose a specific disease entity? Of course not. Instead, it gives us valuable information which is essential in determining not only the current status of the patient, but also the best modes of treatment and when the end result of balance has been obtained.

The understanding and analysis of the biological terrain is as valuable to the doctor and patient as a blood chemistry test. Perhaps even more valuable. In its content, the key can be found to the current underlying dilemma that plagues the patient and also the direction that their body's chemistry must be altered to attain

One out of every three Americans today is diagnosed with a deadly disease.

a balanced biochemical equilibrium.

The biological terrain gives us the key to initiate the proper modes of therapy, to monitor the on-going progress, and to determine when to treat specific symptoms or disease states. It helps us reach down to the core of the patient's imbalance and successfully effect them on a cellular level.

Once your personal biological terrain has been mapped out, whether your mode of treatment is Oriental medicine, herbal, homeopathic, dietary alteration, vitamin and mineral therapy, or even chemotherapeutics, the understanding and analysis of your biological terrain can and must play a primary diagnostic role for most effective body changes to occur. After all, how can you begin a successful body transformation program if you do not know your current state of health and fitness?

The public is saying, "We don't want things that are suppressant. We don't want to take drugs. We want to live naturally. We want to feel better!" We all hear it all the time like a mantra. It doesn't mean that Western doctors aren't dedicated and focused and wonderful; it's just that the public has greater options and should exercise them accordingly.

A state of optimal health is a state of high energy and vitality. Achieving an ideal biological terrain can happen with the aid of natural herbs. Generally, the herbs that boost digestion, elimination, immunity, help create an acid-alkaline balance and increase energy are the most desired. I am a great proponent of herbal remedies and wish to take a closer look at several of the most useful ones on the market today.

Ginkgo: nature's greatest gift?

By now, nearly every person in Western society should know about ginkgo biloba. The ginkgo herb is powerful ammunition used against the destructive forces of aging. Its fantastic ability to aid the circulatory and nervous systems is nothing short of extraordinary.

Ginkgo is believed to be Earth's oldest living tree at 200 million years. The stately ginkgo is more than 100 feet high and eight-feet wide. Also known as the maiden-haired tree, it survived from extinction by individual efforts and was discovered growing freely on China's temple and monastery grounds. Ironically, ginkgo is the only one left in its botanical family and is not closely related to any other known plant. It was a part of the Ginkgoales family, which dates from the Permian period of the Paleozoic era between 225 and 280 million years ago. However, fossils of the bi-lobed leaf have been found in Europe and North America.

Ginkgo was wiped out during the Ice Age some 10,000 years ago. Its therapeutic use has been recorded for the past 4,000 years. Ginkgo extract's medical uses, the Chinese wrote 500 years earlier, included the alleviation of chest problems such as asthma and cough, and was cited for "benefiting the brain." Only now do we know how right they were.

Today, ginkgo is referred to as a "living fossil" and is possibly one of modern medicine's brightest hopes. It is the world's most extensively researched herb. More than 400 chemical, pharmacological, and clinical studies at research centers and universities in Europe and Asia show that ginkgo biloba extract has many important therapeutic uses. Primarily, it increases circulation and oxygenation, particularly to the brain and limbs. This has many vital implications. Ginkgo is one of the most successful substances a person can take to ward off, and to an extent, reverse the effects of aging. French scientists concluded that, "The results confirmed the efficacy of ginkgo extract in cerebral disorders due to aging."

Consistently, studies show that ginkgo can dilate arteries, veins, and capillaries by stimulating peripheral circulation (blood circulation outside the heart muscle itself) and blood flow to the brain. This is why ginkgo is important in the treatment of vascular disorders such as dementia, short-term memory loss, tinnitus (ringing in the ears), headaches, and deteriorating vision. Susceptibility to cold, numbness, and cramping of hands and feet is greatly reduced by the herb. German studies showed that ginkgo can reduce HDL cholesterol levels in 86 percent of the subjects they studied. In other studies, a combination of ginkgo and ginseng herbs reduced blood pressure and prevented abnormal blood clotting.

Long-term use of ginkgo has been documented in the reduction of cardiovascular risk, such as coronary heart disease, hypertension, high cholesterol, and adult onset diabetes.

But what has researchers most excited is ginkgo's effect on the brain. "The management of cerebral edema is one of the unsolved problems in neurology and neurosurgery," said Dr. Ryan Huxtable of the University of Arizona, "but ginkgo extract has proven effective in animal experiments to reduce chemically-induced brain edema. It also protects the liver, reduces arrhythmia, inhibits potentially life-threatening constriction of the bronchi during allergic reactions, and is being evaluated for use in asthma, graft rejection, shock, stroke, organ preservation, and hemodialysis, among other conditions."

No brain disorder appears to affect more people to such a drastic degree as does Alzheimer's disease. It kills more than

100,000 people each year in the United States. Health and Human Services has allocated hundreds of millions of dollars to further study drug development, but this does not include the use of herbs. However, Europeans and Asians have long suspected and documented the effectiveness of ginkgo biloba extract in Alzheimer's sufferers. *The Lancet* reported on the therapeutic success of ginkgo. It stated that a dozen symptoms related to cerebral insufficiency, frequently found among Alzheimer's patients, are alleviated by ginkgo biloba. Such symptoms include difficulty with concentration and memory, absentmindedness, confusion, lack of energy, fatigue, decreased physical performance, depression, anxiety, dizziness, tinnitus, and headaches.

Ginkgo is heavily concentrated with flavanoids, terpenoids, and other substances that make this herb a powerful antioxidant. Simply put, membranes must be fluid so the oxygen and other vital substances can flow freely to the brain and other parts of the body. When the membranes become a bit rusty, so to speak, the adequate supply of nutrients is restricted. This results in the rancidification of fats caused by free radicals. In other words, ginkgo is capable of preventing free radical

The ginkgo herb is powerful ammunition used against the destructive forces of aging.

damage to cellular membranes of the brain, nervous system, and liver. It can even repair lesions in cell membranes that have been damaged by free radicals.

But much of the excitement concerning ginkgo is over its ability to improve circulation and oxygen flow to the brain, which allows it to increase cognitive function and memory. This is important since our brain is particularly sensitive to hypoxia, commonly known as oxygen depravation. Dr. Hans Haas of the Mannheim Clinic in Heidelberg University in Germany said that ginkgo has been shown to increase the brain's tolerance for oxygen deficiency. He says that ginkgo extracts cause a significant increase in the blood flow for those with cerebrovascular disease. But what is quite remarkable about ginkgo is that unlike other drugs designed to improve circulation, natural or synthetic, ginkgo biloba extract increases blood flow not only to healthy areas of the brain, but also to the disease-damaged parts. French researchers discovered, in fact, that those who were severely affected benefited the most from ginkgo.

However, you need not be old or ill in order to reap ginkgo's benefits. In America, it is the young and the health conscious that are discovering and using this potent ancient remedy. The French studied 12 healthy young women and noted improvements in memory and cognitive performance in every one of them. Hence, ginkgo has found itself quite popular among university students and young professionals with demanding careers. In lab studies, rats of various ages increased the number of brain receptors believed to be responsible for memory. The young women studied discovered that their reaction time when undergoing a memory test improved significantly after taking the extract.

In his book, "Mind Food and Smart Pills," Dr. Ross Pelton said, "Ginkgo actually stimulates the release of a substance that relaxes the micro capillaries, thus increasing blood flow. This means that ginkgo may be the most effective remedy known for many of the side effects of aging, such as short-term memory loss, slow thinking and reasoning, dizziness, ringing in the ears, and problems with vertigo and equilibrium."

Ginkgo biloba affects mental alertness by changing the frequency of brain waves. In tests, ginkgo has shown the ability to increase brain alpha rhythms, the brain wave frequencies associated with mental alertness. Improvement in mental alertness becomes evident after only three weeks of ginkgo use and progress continued during a three-month period.

Dr. Willmar Schwabe manufactured the original ginkgo biloba extract in Germany. His company is responsible for sponsoring most of the international research on ginkgo. As ancient as ginkgo's history is, it was only introduced into modern use in 1974. Today, this multi-beneficial herb is prescribed to more than 10 million Europeans annually. It is done so in therapeutic dosages of 40mg of 24 percent ginkgo flavone glycoside extract, three times daily for a total of 120mg. Anything less has simply been proven ineffective consistently. But in the United States, ginkgo is only available in better health food stores as a dietary supplement.

With the tight grip the U.S. pharmaceutical industry has on government regulators and the medical industry in general, ginkgo has not been permitted to see the light of day as it has in Europe and Asia. So far, no drug company has been interested in providing a product to the public that cannot be patented, that they cannot own, and thus not profit from it. Nature has been banned from our pharmacies. The drug efficacy laws were introduced in 1962 and since then, the Food and Drug Administration have allowed not a single new plant medicine on the market.

There is no change of policy in sight. But the public, fed up with allopathic medicine's inability or unwillingness to cure their ills, have sought solutions on their own.

The drug companies, aware of this trend, are thus rushing to develop a patentable, mass marketable synthetic version of a ginkgo substitute but they are finding this process a "living nightmare" according to one industry executive. Although thousands of ginkgo trees are now growing in the Far East, Europe and the United States, the ability to reproduce these chemicals in a laboratory is of vital importance to manufacturers. Now, ginkgolides are being extracted from ginkgo leaves, a most time-consuming process that delivers small amounts of extract from an awful lot of trees.

But to the rescue comes Dr. Elias J. Corey of Harvard University who collected a Nobel Prize in Chemistry for being able to synthesize Ginkgolide B, one of the unique chemical structures that ginkgo leaf extract contains.

The New York Times stated that "British researchers have reported positive results in tests of Ginkgolide B in treating people with asthma and allergic inflammations. Animal studies indicate that the substance might be effective in regulating blood pressure, treating kidney disorders, and counteracting a number of toxins."

But consider the results of other scientific studies when patients were given Ginkgolide B compared to placebos: functional improvement in 65 percent of the patients with arterial leg disease; 100 percent effective in patients with Grade II lower limb arteries (inflammation of an artery); 33 percent effective with sufferers of Raynaud's disease (a spasm of the blood vessels in fingers, toes, etc.); 65 percent v. 13 percent of peripheral pain; 64 percent v. 19 percent improvement from intermittent claudication (poor circulation in the legs); pain attacks in Raynaud's disease patients was 33 percent v. 0 percent.

The Lancet stated that ginkgo extract showed exceptional promise as the drug of choice in the new millennium. What took so long?

Valerian root: Stress-free naturally?

Often, the popular media likes to show photographs of outgoing U.S. presidents and compare them to how they looked when first entering office. The amount of aging that occurs would be staggering. Today, there are few among us who doubt that stress and anxiety are great contributors to premature aging. Being chronically stressed-out is a pretty lousy way to live. As Woody Allen would say, "There are two types of people in this world: the unfortunate and the miserable. The unfortunate are those in truly life-threatening situations, and the rest of us are just miserable."

Whether your stress looms large or small, in chronic dosages it disturbs your

More than 36 million Americans are armed with prescriptions each year for chronic symptoms of anxiety.

physical and emotional well being. The autonomic nervous system is constantly in an aroused state, thus causing epinephrine, norepinephrine, and other hormones to flood the body, resulting in a rapid heart rate, dilation of the pupils, and increased flow of blood to the muscles. Thus, the daily lugging of worry, fear, and anger usually results in aching muscles, sleepless nights, stomach upsets, skin breakouts, and a number of other conditions from mild to deadly serious.

At times, to ease the discomforts of stress, we turn to medications—from over the counter sleeping pills and painkillers to heavy-duty prescription benzodiazepine drugs like Valium and Xanax. More than 36 million Americans are armed with such prescriptions each year for chronic symptoms of anxiety. The side effect of these drugs can be serious and within a month of regular use, one can become addicted. Withdrawal has been known to be difficult at best and fatal at worst.

But medicinal herbs can in many cases calm the nerves, reduce the tension, ease insomnia and reduce pain like chemical drugs do, but without the dangers and often with additional benefits. Herbs are not addictive and some actually nourish and strengthen the nervous system.

To treat anxiety, valerian, hops, passion flower, scullcap, chamomile, and lemon balm are often used, but I wish to focus on the curative powers of valerian root here specifically.

Valerian root was greatly favored by Arab physicians. It found its way to Europe and was frequently prescribed for depression, insomnia, migraines, menstrual cramps, and even epilepsy. During World War I, soldiers were given valerian root for shell shock. This herb is well documented for the relief of anxiety and insomnia. Unlike sleeping pills, which are actually antihistamines and are generally not effective after a few nights of usage since your body develops tolerance, valerian root does not create the side effects of dry mouth, constipation, and dizziness as do over-the-counter sleeping pills. You are also not left groggy in the morning.

Valerian root is believed to be most extraordinary for the sedative effect it has on the central nervous system. One particular study found valerian an effective sedative for agitated patients while it stimulates those afflicted with fatigue. The herb is not only terrific for insomnia, but is a superb remedy for anxiety, nervous tension, and headaches. Little known, but equally impressive, is valerian's strengthening action on the heart. It controls palpitations and lowers blood pressure.

Valerian is further used for nervous dyspepsia, stomach and menstrual cramps and for a spastic or irritable bowel. Since toxins from synthetic drugs are very dangerous and an anxiety-filled life is not a fair trade for early aging, valerian root is a safe alternative for those times when we need intervention in stress control.

Echinacea and Astragalus: the world's best immune system enhancers?

One of the best deterrents to premature aging is a strong immune system. Vitality and high energy, the hallmark of youth, are byproducts of robust health, which is not possible when your immune system is weakened.

For centuries, Native Americans were aware of the health boosting powers of this purple cone flower. More than a dozen tribes relied on the several species of Echinacea. By the early 1900s, the extract of E. purpurea was the leading herb sold in the United States. But soon, allopathy (medicine as we know it today) was established as the standard medicine with its reliance on synthetic, chemical "wonder drugs" and Echinacea was booted out of favor. The Germans, however, felt differently. From the early 1930s, it has become the medicine of choice among many Europeans for treating infection. After extensive research by the Germans showed Echinacea to be a powerful and effective immune builder and a safe antibiotic, the health-conscience Americans once again began drinking Echinacea tea and swallowing Echinacea drops and tablets that they purchased in local health food stores.

But most American doctors are unaware of this natural immunity booster and no pharmacy stocks a single drug with Echinacea in it. After all, in 1910, the American Medical Association declared it useless! But the Europeans aren't impressed with such a declaration and rightfully so. More than 140 Echinacea products are available to the German public today. They include tinctures, salves for sores and wounds, liquid extracts, capsules, teas, and injections for fast acting results, among other forms.

More than 350 scientific studies document Echinacea's effect on the body. This herb is a non-specific immunostimulant, meaning it generally conditions and strengthens the immune system overall and doesn't target a particular organism.

In lab studies, Echinacea has been able to improve the immune system in many ways. The herb is able to increase the number of immune system cells. It further helps develop cells within the bone marrow and lymphatic tissue, and speeds their development into immunocompetent or functioning immune cells. It speeds their release into circulation, so more are present in the blood and the lymph, while it improves their activity, as measured by the rate of phagocytosis. Simply stated, it makes cells that are responsible for warding off invading organisms work much better. Furthermore, Echinacea increases the production of chemicals in the immune system like interferon, interleukins, and the tumor necrosis factor. In addition, Echinacea prevents an enzyme known as gyaluronidase that bacteria rely on to enter the body cells and result in infection. This inhabitation also aids with wound healing by stimulating new tissue formation.

"A well known and much utilized effect of Echinacea is the promotion of wound healing, especially old wounds and ulcers that refuse to heal," said Dr. Weiss in his hugely successful, *Weiss' Herbal Medicine*. He added that given internally, the cone flower Echinacea builds resistance and stimulates both the lymphatic vascular system and the fibroblasts. It has been proven a useful drug in improving the body's own resistance in infectious conditions of all kinds, particularly influenza and colds. Echinacea is taken as soon as influenza-type symptoms appear. Small doses frequently repeated will be adequate every two or three hours on the first and second day following an infection.

Known as *the great herbal convincer*, today Echinacea is used by millions of Europeans and their physicians. Americans are coming around slowly, basically due to word of mouth and alternative health literature. It has definitely been determined that Echinacea preparations have a solid track record in clinical and laboratory studies, and thousands of doctors currently prescribe them for a long list of infectious diseases.

"We are on the threshold of a new era of natural products research, said Steven Foster, a prolific writer on Echinacea. "The negative vestiges of bygone antagonisms should give rise to new applications of herbal medicine to public health care. A rational change in our drug laws is essential. When viewed with objectivity and an open, inquiring mind, Echinacea symbolizes the potential of new herbalism, where science can be blended to produce positive results."

Today, we face antibiotic-resistant bacteria due to antibiotic abuse in grave proportions. As the "magic bullet" or "wonder drug" dream fizzles, Echinacea is an idea whose time has finally come—again.

Echinacea, although among the most studied of herbs for its positive effect on the immune system, is not the only one that can achieve this great accomplishment. The ancient Chinese employed astragalus to boost immunity and today scientific research shows them to have been incredibly accurate. Traditional Chinese Medicine claims that astragalus helps put the body's energy in balance. The herb has long been believed to protect the body against disease by increasing resistance.

Astragalus acts as a powerful stimulant to our immune system by causing an increase in the quantity and activity of immune cells all through the body. This heightened immune action eliminates foreign particles (by phagocytosis) after 35 days of astragalus use. But most remarkable was the herb's effect on cancer victims. Consistently, scientific studies showed that astragalus extracts can restore the function of damaged immune cells taken from cancer patients. Researchers said that, "a complete immune restoration can be achieved by using a fractionated extract of astragalus membranaceus...." Herbalists prescribe astragalus to ward off colds and infectious disease. After all, studies showed that the herb reduced incidence of common colds among users and shortened the duration of colds by nearly half.

Reishi: the longevity herb?

The healing powers of certain herbs are plentiful and these days as so much is being focused on immunity, scientists have taken to exploring Reishi as well. Reishi contributes to a longer life by strengthening the immune system and by controlling free radicals. Korean scientists have found that the Reishi herb hardens muscles of the immune system by super-charging two types of fighting cells: macrophages and polymor phonuclear leukocytes. But perhaps the most promising aspect of Reishi power is its effect on cancer. The Linus Pauling Institute of Science and Medicine found that Reishi has great prom-ise for managing cancer, particularly when teamed with megadoses of vitamin C daily. He believes that reishi shows even greater promise in cancer prevention.

> Reishi con-tributes to a longer life by strengthening the immune system and by controlling free radicals.

Reishi is a rare mushroom that Westerners began to use only two decades ago. In China, it is also called Ganoderma, ling-chih-tsao, and wu-ling-chih. It's a tough wood-like mushroom, which consists of more than 90 percent indigestible fiber.

For more than a thousand years, the Chinese relied on Reishi for disease prevention and healing. In Asia today, it is used for regulating blood pressure, pre-venting abnormal blood clotting, strengthening the heart, cleansing the blood, detoxifying and regenerating the liver, overcoming insomnia, kidney prob-lems, managing allergies, but perhaps most importantly, combating free radicals and supporting the immune system.

Chinese doctors appreciated Reishi's effect on "the knotted and tight chest." Today, doctors confirm that in lab experiments, erratic electrocardiograms of animals with heart disease returned to normal after Reishi extract was injected.

Tokyo university researchers studied patients with essential (inherited) high blood pressure. They gave 240mg of Reishi daily to for six months and found that the patients had normal blood pressure.

In Moscow, scientists were on a mission to discover herbs that aided the heart. At the Cardiology Research Center at the Academy of Medical Sciences, researchers studied 21 herbs to discover which most effectively prevented and cured the buildup of atherosclerotic plaque in the arteries. They concluded that for prevention and therapy, two mushrooms withstood the rigorous testing: Reishi and shitake.

Other scientists have reported that Reishi actually reversed the toxic effects of carbon tetrachloride and ethionine in the livers, minimizing the fatty condition that has so frequently led to cirrhosis of the liver. Then, quite by accident, researchers discovered that Reishi acts as a mild sedative. While patients were being treated for other conditions, doctors realized they always relaxed and mellowed out. Later, when tested against insomnia, it was effective without causing any side effects.

Reishi has also been shown to control all four major types of allergic reaction, including chronic bronchitis, asthma, contact dermatitis, as well as the garden variety of sneezes, wheezes, itches, and stuffy nose.

Chinese hospitals have given Reishi formula to 2,000 patients with chronic bronchitis, a tough one to handle. They had great results in 60-90 percent of the cases. After a mere four months, bronchitis sufferers had an increase of immunoglobulin A, the leading immune system protector in the respiratory tract. People who lack immunoglobulin almost always suffer from severe allergies.

Garlic: the currency of every millennium

From the purple cone flower to a wood-like mushroom to a humble clove of garlic, these are some of nature's greatest gifts to us all. Yet they still go underutilized and under appreciated. Let's take a closer look at garlic. It boasts a medical history more solid than just about any other substance known to man. Far from being the latest "health food," garlic has kept its power for more than 6,000 years. Although garlic has only recently been thoroughly studied and accepted as the ideal food, its history is rich and powerful indeed.

When the tomb of King Tut was discovered, it contained garlic bulbs—dried and perfectly preserved. The great pyramid of Cheops of Giza could be completed only after rations of garlic were increased as demanded by the workers. At today's cost, that was an extra expense of more than $2 million. When King Nabonidus lost the throne of Babylon to Cyrus in 538 B.C., he had to transfer his wealth—more than 150,000 strings of garlic! That's some 15,000,000 bulbs.

The Greeks understood that garlic was a source of vibrant health and energy period. Aristotle said it was a tonic to invigorate every cell and restore health. Hippocrates prescribed garlic for "increasing the flow of urine, relaxing the stomach, and aiding a cough with pus or signs of suppuration in a sick man." Today, we refer to it as a diuretic, digestive aid, and antibiotic. Dioscorides, the most influential writer of Roman times, confirmed the same uses as well as finding garlic an excellent antiparasitic and anticongestant that also relieves bronchitis and lowers blood fats and cholesterol.

In ancient times, garlic was used for the same reasons we use it today, they merely didn't have the medical jargon and clinical studies to prove it. In the past two decades, more than 800 papers have been published on the benefits of garlic.

Garlic has a strong reputation for combating bacterial diseases like throat and ear infections, stomach upsets, diarrhea, bronchitis, infected wounds, and sinus problems. In clinical studies, garlic has often outperformed accepted antibiotics in standard culture dish tests. In fact, it has a broad-spectrum action against various virulent bacteria. Garlic consumed on a daily basis is known to keep infection at bay in the first place. When garlic is increased at the onset of an infection, it can prevent it from becoming a full-blown disease.

Unlike antibiotics, bacterial resistance to garlic cannot happen. Needless to say, there are no side effects as with prescription drugs. In the 1950s, 100,000 units of penicillin were considered a serious dose. Today, several million is hardly unusual.

Garlic has been used on respiratory ailments so successfully that a license was issued for garlic by the Ministry of Health in the United Kingdom that allows garlic product manufacturers to claim it is a remedy used for the treatment of rhinitis (inflammation of the nasal membranes) and catarrh (throat and bronchial tubes).

Garlic is also a known anti-fungal. It can slow down or kill some 60 fungi and more than 20 types of bacteria—including some bacteria that have become resistant to antibiotics. A component in garlic, allicin, kills candida, a fungal overgrowth usually a result of antibiotic use. It is now the leading natural treatment for candida.

Garlic enhances the immune response and thus is effective against viral infections. It causes the production of more T-killer cells in the blood. T-killer cells attack virus-loaded cells and cancer cells.

Heart and circulatory diseases are the leading cause of death in Western society. Half of all deaths fall in this category. Garlic can improve all the factors leading to such disease: high cholesterol, low HDL cholesterol, high blood pressure, edema, and blood that clots too rapidly.

Garlic is a potent antioxidant. Deadly free radicals can alter our cells' vital DNA. Once the DNA is altered, the cell is ready for cancer. Garlic can inhibit cancer formation and growth. Researchers at Pennsylvania State University found that garlic powder can reduce the incidence of breast cancer in mice that were fed a cancer-causing chemical by 70-90 percent. Scientists at Loma Linda University concluded that, "Garlic interferes with the transformation of normal cells into cancer cells." Garlic is most effective against stomach, nose, throat, lymphatic, rectal, colon, breast, and esophageal cancers. The National Cancer Institute has funded a $20 million series of

> Garlic boasts a medical history more solid than just about any other substance known to man...
>
> Unlike antibiotics, bacterial resistance to garlic cannot happen.

studies to examine the anticancer effects of several herbs, especially garlic.

Garlic is incredibly beneficial to our overall health because a single clove has some 70 sulfur-containing oils, carbohydrates, protein, fiber, vitamin A, B1, B2, B3, C, zinc, calcium, manganese, germanium, selenium, copper, iron, and a nucleic acid, adenosine, which is a building block of DNA and RNA.

Natural organic garlic in its raw form is considered the most effective medicinally. But due to its socially unacceptable odor, you can turn to a processed form IF it is the cool-dried method. This dry powder contains all the beneficial properties of raw garlic—other forms of processing do not.

One or two cloves a day, or its equivalent in garlic powder, is the required dose for prevention of circulatory problems. But for antibacterial and other therapeutic uses, take 3-6 cloves daily.

Throughout history, every culture on earth has relied on herbs and plants to maintain health, cure disease, slow down the aging process, and prolong life. The Sumerians left behind clay tablets from around 4,000 B.C., showing that they had apothecaries for dispensing medicinal herbs.

A Chinese book from 3,000 B.C., *The Pen Tsao*, listed 1,000 herb formulas that had been used for thousands of years prior. British settlers who landed in Plymouth in 1630 planted herb gardens almost immediately. As I already mentioned, Native Americans were well aware of the healing powers of plants, having cultivated Echinacea and goldenseal among others.

Today, many mainstream people have claimed that mainstream medicine has failed them. Young adults have seen terrible conditions and fatal diseases destroy the lives of their parents and grandparents. Almost in unison, they are saying, "Not us! There's got to be a better way." Hence, collectively we are realizing that a weakened immune system is the cause of most preventable suffering—the destroyer of the good life. At last, again, we are turning to safer, more effective treatment and realizing that prevention is the only true way to good health and a long, happy, and productive life.

Stevia: The sweetest thing of all

It's 250-400 times sweeter than sugar, contains no calories and has no ill effects when consumed. In fact, it is safe for diabetics. So where has stevia been for centuries? In Paraguay. And now it is virtually found all over the world, although commercial producers of aspartame particularly, and the artificial sweeteners industry in general, has placed tremendous pressure on the FDA to ban stevia as an "unapproved food additive." Therefore, this all natural and safe sugar substitute can only be labeled as a "dietary supplement" and purchased retail at health food stores and whole foods stores.

Stevia came a long way in the United States from being an "import alert" to the most healthy sugar alternative on the market today. The humble herb is a shrub belonging to the sunflower family of plants and is native to the northern regions of South America. It is found in the wild in

> Stevia is 250-400 times sweeter than sugar, contains no calories, and has no ill effects when consumed.

semi-arid habitats ranging from grassland to mountain terrain. It is grown commercially in Brazil, Central America, Israel, Thailand, China, and the United States. Stevia's leaves contain chemicals called glycosides, which produces its sweetness. The Brazilians used it for centuries as a sweetener in yerba mate and other medicinal teas for treating conditions such as obesity, high blood pressure, and heartburn. It has recently been the focus of attention thanks to the low-carb, low-sugar diets.

Since 1977, stevia and its extracts have captured more than 40 percent of the Japanese market. They began cultivating stevia as an alternative to artificial sweeteners like cyclamate and saccharin, which were suspected carcinogens. Stevia sweeteners are widely used in food products, soft drinks, and for table use.

But the United States and its sugar and substitute sugar industry is still engaged in protectionists' agendas while stevia is placed as a fringe product for health nuts in select stores. In 1991, at the request of an aspartame manufacturer, the FDA labeled stevia as an "unsafe food additive" and restricted its importation. In 1995, the FDA revised its stance to permit stevia to be sold as a "dietary supplement." As Rob McCaleb, the president and founder of the Herb Research Foundation stated, "Sweetness is big money. Nobody wants to see something cheap and easy to grow on the market competing with the things they worked so hard to get approved."

Stevia is primarily sold as a powder or liquid but there are some differences; not all stevia extract powders are the same. The taste, sweetness and cost of the available white stevia powders depend on their degree of refinement and the quality of the stevia plant used. Some powders have an aftertaste while others don't, so you may wish to experiment with different brands.

The liquid also comes in several forms. There is the dark syrupy black liquid that comes from boiling the leaves, while steeping stevia leaves in distilled water and grain alcohol is also popular. A third alternative is a liquid made from the white powder concentrate mixed with water and preserved in grape-seed extract.

Either way, it's an absolute Godsend for those of us who enjoy the sweet taste but not the bitter results of sugar or artificial sweeteners.

A suggested meal plan to increase your energy:

<u>On rising:</u>
Drink a glass of spring water with a rounded teaspoon of acidophilus.
Take digestive enzymes before each meal.

<u>Breakfast:</u>
Fresh fruit in season and a glass of fresh carrot juice with ginger, bee pollen, and bee propolis. Wait half an hour and then have a hot whole grain cereal or whole grain toast with kefir cheese or eggs.
Supplements: vitamin C, vitamin E, vitamins B-complex, a multi vitamin-mineral, and germanium.

<u>Mid-morning:</u>
Cup of hot potassium broth or a vegetable juice. Siberian ginseng* and hawthorn berry** extract in small amount of room temperature water.
<u>Lunch:</u>
Brown or basmati rice with fish or seafood, or organic chicken or tofu and steamed vegetables or green salad; or beans or lentils with brown rice and a mix of vegetables. Cup of green tea.
Supplements: vitamin C, vitamins B-complex, co-enzyme Q10, Kyolic garlic.***

---

* Siberian ginseng is a long-term tonic that supports the adrenal glands.

** Hawthorn berry dilates coronary blood vessels, lowers cholesterol levels, and restores heart muscle. It increases vitamin C levels. Hawthorn berry is useful for anemia, cardiovascular and circulatory disorders, high cholesterol, and lowered immunity.

*** Kyolic garlic can be substituted for fresh garlic if you choose not to be offensive with garlic odor.

Mid-afternoon:

Fresh fruit in season or a crunchy vegetable. Spirulina and gink-go biloba extract.

Dinner:

A whole grain food of your choice and legumes with vegetables and a green salad with nuts, seeds, and sprouts.**** A cup of alfal-fa tea.

Supplements: vitamin C, vitamin E, multi vitamin-mineral, evening primrose oil, and Kyolic garlic.

Bedtime:

Chamomile tea with fresh lemon.

**** *Sprouts can be alfalfa, red clover, mung bean, radish or sunflower. They are highly nutritious and a great source of protein in the form of amino acids, chlorophyll, enzymes and plant hormones. A good source of vitamins A, C, B-complex and E, with balanced minerals and trace minerals. Be sure all sprouts are organically grown.*

CHAPTER 11
ENDURANCE, STRENGTH AND
FLEXIBILITY TRANSFORMATION

If you have been following the advice given thus far, by now you are eating well and changes are taking place within your body that will immensely influence your well being if you stay with the program. At this point, you can boost your diet with more protein and even higher concentrations of nutrients because now you are ready to really focus on your body with greater physical activity.

Endurance and strength is nutrition coupled with aerobic activity and strength training. After all, when we gain control over our bodies, we gain control over our lives. Yet so many of us are still missing out. By now, we all know that in addition to vital dietary changes, we require aerobic activity, but so few of us fully understand why or how to effectively achieve this goal. Aerobic exercise, like the term "free radicals" are words we have all heard and think we know what they mean, but we aren't sure of the precise definition or of its benefits or dangers.

Aerobic capacity is simply defined as how well the heart and lungs bring oxygen to the muscles and how efficiently the muscles then use the oxygen to generate energy during sustained exercise, which drops by as much as 10 percent per decade after the age of 25. But the latest research from NASA/Johnson Space Center and the Institute of Aerobic Research in Dallas indicates that even this decline can be prevented. Their studies confirm previous estimates by experts who claimed that much of the functional losses that set in between the ages of 30 and 70 are in fact attributed to lack of exercise.

They discovered that half of the "age-related" decline in aerobic power was actually due NOT to age per se, but to changes in body composition—namely, an increased percentage of body fat—and decreased physical activity. These two factors interact, of course: those who exercise regularly tend to be lean. In fact, lean active older people tend to be much fitter aerobically than younger people who are less active or have more body fat. For instance, if the average 30-year-old increases his percentage of body fat by 50 percent and becomes sedentary, which is the typical scenario, *choice* not *aging* has virtually everything to do with how healthy we look and feel throughout our entire life.

Aerobic exercise is any form of physical exercise that requires additional effort by the heart and lungs to meet the increased demand for oxygen from the skeletal muscles. The exercise

> Much of the functional losses that set in between the ages of 30 and 70 are, in fact, attributed to lack of exercise.

requires heavier breathing than passive muscular activity and results in increased heart and lung efficiency, with a minimum of wasted energy.

To be fit is to have a strong lean body, muscular endurance, a healthy heart, and lungs and lots of energy. Aerobic exercise works the whole body, therefore benefiting the whole body. After a good work out, you feel as if you have more energy because exercising aerobically makes you use more energy. Consequently, you usually feel less tired throughout the day and generally have energy left over for other activities without feeling exhausted by the end of the day.

When you are both sedentary and under mental stress, adrenaline builds up in your heart and brain. As a result, when you become exhausted, your entire system is loaded with adrenaline. The best way to counteract such as effect is with aerobic exercise, which will revive and revitalize you all over again. When your body is given the opportunity to process and deliver oxygen rapidly and efficiently, you will naturally have more potent vitality and energy.

Yet, as I have stated throughout this book, most of us don't care for exercise—at least not enough to do something about it. The United States President's Council on Physical Fitness says that 95 percent of Americans are not in shape. So much for the 1980s aerobics revolution!

The same can be said for the British. Today, an average 20-year-old man has the body capacity of a 40-year-old: he cannot climb a flight of stairs or run a city block without exhaustion. Thus it is quite true when we hear it said that a man does not die, he kills himself! But conditioning the cardiovascular and pulmonary system—the heart, blood vessels, and lungs can change all that. Aerobic exercise can transform your body through endurance activities of greater intensity and duration than you are already used to at present.

Regular exercise does more for the heart than any other activity. It strengthens the heart muscle, decreases blood pressure, reduces heart rate, lowers blood cholesterol and triglycerides, reduces the likelihood of developing an irregular heartbeat and improves collateral circulation (when new blood vessels form to take over the circulation of blocked vessels).

Thus, not only does aerobic exercise make us healthier and fitter, we *feel* better and now the latest research tells us that it can help us get smarter as well. Aerobic exercise does more than elevate the heart rate and make us break into a sweat. It lifts our spirit and boosts self-esteem. Nearly a decade ago, some of America's leading brain researchers held a first time ever symposium in Chicago to discuss the connection between physical movement and learning. Since then, research has reaffirmed their findings. According to experts, the greater confidence, as reported by so many aerobic exercise enthusiasts, is not mere fancy. Something far more complex is happening here. They suggest that in much the same way that exercise shapes up the bones,

Today, an average 20-year-old man has the body capacity of a 40-year-old.

muscles, heart, and lungs, it also strengthens the basal ganglia, cerebellum, and corpus callosum—deep innards of the brain. Thus, what is good for the heart is also good for the brain!

Hence, exercise not only fuels the brain with a better blood supply but it feeds brain cells with a heartier supply of natural substances, known as neurotrophins, that enhance their growth. Add to the aerobics a series of complex coordinated movements like dance moves, and the brain produces a greater number of connections between its neurons.

The documented benefits of aerobic exercise are vast indeed: decreases the risk of heart disease and stroke, lowers blood pressure, reduces stress and tension, increases the good cholesterol while lowering the bad cholesterol, lessens the incidence of colon cancer, the list goes on and on. Aerobic exercise burns calories and promotes fat loss, retards the rate of bone loss in older people and helps prevent adult-onset diabetes.

Any act of physical activity is welcomed, since 60 percent of Americans do not engage in virtually any leisure-time physical activity. However, only exercise that is of intense, aerobic quality for a minimum of 20 to 30 minutes three times a week, combined with regular strength training, will actually transform your body and extend your life.

Generally, it takes about one-and-a-half months of an hour of aerobic exercise three to four times a week before a firmer body and fewer inches are noticeable. Weight loss will occur if you combine the body transformation dietary recommendations and strength training with aerobics. A good aerobic hour can burn around 600 calories. This is equivalent to a seven-mile jog. A marvelous bonus is that you continue to burn calories at twice your normal rate *after* you stop exercising. Up to six hours later, in fact. While you are watching TV, reading, eating or sleeping, you are still burning calories at twice your normal rate.

Soon, as you become more fit, your body will demand a greater volume of oxygen over a longer period of time. As your body is transforming, you will be able to work harder and longer without shortness of breath and a loss of energy. Additionally, as your body becomes far more efficient and finely tuned, you will recover in no time at all after a vigorous session and will have a greater stamina throughout the day. Furthermore, you will benefit from improved circulation that will not only contribute to healthier organs, but a better complexion. Finally, you will improve your flexibility, balance, coordination, and body control overall, which will be evident in your everyday life.

Therefore, it is no secret that the most fit people tend to live the longest. But what may be surprising to hear is that the biggest jump in life expectancy occurs for people who go from being totally sedentary to being moderately active. And although life expectancy is desirable, quality of life is preferred. This is where exercise, if it could be sold as a product, would be a trillion dollar industry. Unfortunately, most of us discover the full power of exercise by necessity and not choice.

It was through necessity and not choice that I rediscovered exercise in a major way. About a decade ago, the unthinkable happened: I suffered an excruciating persistent backache that was making my life miserable. Being quite certain that it was a serious medical crisis that required immediate physical intervention I headed to a top hospital to see one of America's leading orthopedic surgeons. Further, I requested that two other orthopedists be present to examine the x-rays and my physical condition. They waited in their white doctors' smocks and hound dog expressions as I arrived. I was terrified and expected the worst news. In hindsight, perhaps my actions were a tad drastic. But 20-somethings and 30-somethings just don't suffer from debilitating backaches! Or so I thought. The good doctor tried to keep a straight face as he put me through paces that might challenge a Laker's cheerleader, but which I was able to perform without too much difficulty. After I explained my history to him, current lack of physical activity and high levels of stress, he repeated it all back to me and advised me to exercise more and stress less. This medical advice set me back nearly $10,000. He told me to begin by walking and stretching and to reduce my stress level. He said that if this approach didn't work, he hoped that I had really good insurance, because it was going to get very costly. I decided to walk...and nobody has been able to stop me since. In fact, to this day, I walk ten miles a day, five to six days a week. That's a walk from Phoenix to Palm Springs every month. In fact, over the years, I figured that I could have walked about halfway to China by now. Backaches, I am happy to report, are a thing of the past.

I did learn, however, that 80 percent of all Americans suffer from backaches and that *inactivity* is considered a national health crisis. I began by rising at the first crow of the rooster. I'd slip into my sweats and Nike's only to discover that I was the only civilian stalking the earth at such an hour along the golf course in the Arizona desert. These walks allowed me to reconnect with nature, see the morning dew on blades of grass, hear the birds sing, feed the ducks on the ponds, and have quiet time to think. These are things I always enjoyed in the past, but somehow along the way, my work became all consuming, and like so many of us, I just became too busy and oblivious to engage in what I began to consider self-indulging rituals. I couldn't have been more wrong.

The good old ordinary act of normal walking has been shown to provide most of the benefits that runners achieve but without the knee, hamstring, and back problems.

Occasionally, I would run into a few geriatric types strolling with the dog or the odd parrot. In no time at all it seemed, my walks became more and more brisk and I would clock in 8-12 miles a day. I discovered that my mood lifted, energy level went up and stress was manageable. At times, the wise-guy golfer would cruise up in a cart and say that he's been watching me for days and was just wondering, "Where are you going?" I'd pick up a stray golf ball, hold it out in his direction and reply, "I think I have one of your balls."

Walking in the 1990s had become a *new* fitness frenzy! Today, there are even magazines devoted to walking. This type of aerobic activity has been more than just exercise and that's perhaps one of the main reasons that people stick with it. I mean, you can tell who's on a leisurely stroll, who is engaged in a quality time walk and talk, or who is burning off steam at the end of a hectic day.

Walking soon became a therapeutic experience more than exercise to me. As I would let my mind go free and wander, it would usually come up with creative solutions to problems. I'd also come up with new ideas as well as mentally prioritize and organize what I needed to do at the time. It was the time to focus. As it turned out, the physical benefits were a welcomed side effect.

I must confess, however, it wasn't without doubt that I began this "new exercise program." Walking? Yeah, right. But I had no choice, for my back pain would not allow me to do much else. I bought into a common prejudice: old people walk, young people run. The activity just didn't seem to demand enough effort for me to believe that it could keep me fit. I was wrong. Although we still need to incorporate other types of exercise into our fitness regime, walking is a safe, easy and fun long-term exercise. As of late, people seem to be catching on to this, since the latest surveys show that nearly a third of Americans now walk specifically for health and fitness, up from barely a fourth less than a decade ago.

These regular walkers discovered what I discovered as well—that walking helps elevate the mood, lessen tension, ease confusion, boost self-esteem, increase energy and strengthen the body. Metabolism increases. Heart rate decreases. Breathing increases. Muscle tension is reduced. There are changes in hormones and in brain neurotransmitters which have a positive influence on thinking and mood.

The good old ordinary act of normal walking has been shown to provide most of the benefits that runners achieve but without the knee, hamstring, and back problems. We all hear about the *runner's high*, but walking can do wonders for the mood as well. We know that the mind affects the body, but now we understand that the body affects the mind as well. A brisk 20-40 minute walk every day can tremendously improve emotional stability, according to research at Indiana State University. Those scientists concluded that the psychological benefits of exercise like walking are comparable to gains from standard types of psychotherapy.

When depressed individuals were assigned an exercise, relaxation therapy or psychotherapy, researchers found that after 12 weeks all three activities reduced depression, but nearly a year later, the depression of those who had chosen exercise and relaxation techniques showed the greatest improvement, while the psychotherapy groups did not fare as well. Experts say that regular exercise provides us with a sense of control over our bodies, allowing us to feel better about ourselves overall—to feel literally transformed.

The fastest way to boost the immune system is to take a good walk, according to researchers at Loma Linda University School of Public Health. When sedentary people take up walking for 45 minutes every day, after about three months the levels of antibodies, which help combat infection increase by some 20 percent. When they did come down with a cold or flu, their ailments lasted less than half as long as those of sedentary people.

Physically active women are also far better at managing the symptoms of premenstrual syndrome (PMS). When a group of PMS sufferers were put on a walking program, scientists at Indiana's Ball State University found that after only four months, the women reported a significant reduction in PMS symptoms, mainly the absence of mood swings, increased appetite, and crying spells, but also a reduction in anxiety, breast tenderness, cravings for sweets, and fluid retention. The researchers concluded that the anti-PMS effect of regular exercise is probably due to an increase in the levels of endorphins, the chemical messengers in the brain that produce a feeling of well being. But all of this aside, what society appears to be most obsessed about today is weight loss. Although being overweight is an epidemic with no end in sight, dieting is NOT the answer. Fortunately, after a mere ten weeks of daily walking, body fat can be reduced without any special diet, reports the Journal of the American Dietetic Association. Simply by walking a few hours a week, you can trim inches from your measurements without necessarily losing any weight. Researchers at Baylor University compared dieters to walkers and found that dieters had initially lost weight quickly, but had gained most of it right back. The walkers, on the other hand had taken a longer time to lose weight, but the loss was steady and permanent.

Since your entire body atrophies if your walking muscles atrophy, it is simple enough to assume that walking aerobically is one of the greatest forms of exercise. After all, more muscles are used when walking than during just about any other type of activity. You simultaneously improve your leg and thigh muscles, abdominals, and buttocks. Walking works the shoulders, triceps, and forearms. Even your skin improves, making it stronger, thicker, and more elastic. In addition, most sports and other physical activities tend to develop only certain groups of muscles, thus leaving you physically unbalanced. Walking develops all muscles equally. Initially, your goal should be to increase your mileage gradually each day and to walk aerobically for a set time and set distance. In addition to set walking times, you can increase the amount of walking you do each day by walking to and from work and appointments as much as possible, take the stairs as opposed to the elevator, walk to do your errands and incorporate lunch-time walks and evening strolls into your day. A friend who is an agent in the entertainment industry makes a point of strolling across his office for hours while on the phone with a headset. He rarely sits down while conducting his daily business. It is a creative solution to a lower back, shoulder, and neck pain problem that he developed after two years with a telephone jammed between his jaw and shoulder.

Your aerobic walk should consist of 20-30 minutes at 4-5 miles per hour, 3-5 times per week. This can be very easily achieved on a treadmill if you're in the city, but many people prefer doing it in the outdoor air. If certain days present obstacles to your walking routine, you can certainly make up for the shortfall later on or over the weekend. If you incorporate a long weekend walk or hike, you are well on your way to better health and a better body. The key is to be consciously aware of how sedentary you have become so that you can do something about it before inactivity manifests itself undesirably. Commitment, action, and consistency are what will lead you to the body transformation that you desire.

Aerobic activity is so important because it promotes cardiorespiratory fitness—the health and function of the heart, lungs, and circulatory system. When working out aerobically, you require more than the normal consumption of oxygen. Again, aerobic simply means working with oxygen. To many people still, it seems that when we hear the word "aerobic," we tend to think of a room full of skimpily-clad bodies all moving in time to very up-beat music. Of course, there are a number of activities that are aerobic. These include walking, jogging, running, step and aerobic classes, swimming, cycling, rowing, hiking, racquet sports, and naturally, step and aerobic classes. When you work out aerobically, that main fuel comes from fat, along with carbohydrates, so it forces the fat cells to release fat. By doing this on a regular basis, your fat releasing enzyme, HSL, is forced to release fat and in turn, your fat cells are going to decrease.

Benefits of aerobic fitness:
- Decreased body fat stores.
- Decreased total cholesterol.
- Decreased symptoms of depression, anxiety and tension.
- Increased heart function.
- Reduction in blood pressure.
- Decreased resting heart rate.
- Increased blood flow to activate muscles.
- Increased lung capacity.
- Increased mobilization and utilization of fat.

Exercise selection:

Since many of you are reading this book to find out how to transform your body inside and out, the aim is to give you recommendations that will help you along with your personal goals. Obviously, you have to be able to take on the activity of your choice. It is no use deciding that you will go cycling 10 miles every other day if you have dodgy knees. Likewise, you would not choose swimming if you still use arm floats. So, be realistic about what you are capable of doing.

Next, you need to look at your available time. If you spend two hours commuting every day, then there is no point in joining a local gym where you live, because chances are you will never get there. On the other hand, if you do have a couple of hours every day, by all means go to the gym. Many people have found that having a personal trainer is time efficient, disciplined, and more of a necessity than a luxury. It is important in the long run that you select an activity that you will enjoy. There is no point is doing something that holds no interest for you.

Finally, you will need to decide whether your chosen activity requires equipment or facilities. Most health clubs will have all the aerobics facilities available and many have swimming pools and racquet courts. Most aerobic activities require little or no equipment at all. Often it is better to start out this way and then invest time and money when you are convinced that you want to continue.

Cross-country skiing and squash are rated as the top calorie burners. As cross-country skiing is not readily available to everyone, a machine that goes through the same motions is the next best thing. Hill climbing is another huge energy user. An eight-hour day with brief rests will burn an average of 4,000 calories. Swimming is also a fantastic calorie-burning exercise, more so for men than women, unfortunately. This is mainly due to the fact that women's higher fat content makes them more buoyant, whereas men have greater effort staying afloat and pushing their bodies through the water. Nevertheless, it's still a great way to get your aerobic exercise.

My personal recommendation for an aerobic activity would be one in which exercise intensity is easily sustained with little variability in the heart rate: walking, jogging, running, aerobic dancing or step aerobics, cross-country skiing, and the various aerobic machines on offer in the

As exercise intensity increases, so does the overall rate at which all calories are burned —whether they are carbohydrates or fats.

fitness clubs. These are all activities that you can pretty much get out there and complete within 45 minutes. My second choice would be soccer, basketball, racquetball, choreographed dance routines, and so forth, where the activities are variable in intensity. These should be done more for recreation on alternative days when you cannot do the first group of recommended aerobic activities.

Exercise duration:

Over the past decade, the duration of aerobic activity has been a subject of debate and we have seen quite a number of changes being made in this area. Initially, the guidelines were to do 20 minutes of aerobic work three times per week for the most effective way to burn fat or increase your lean body tissue (fat-free mass). Then more research came out stating that we need to increase the duration of the aerobic activity from 30-45 minutes three times per week. This was overwhelming or simply too much for most people. As a result, they gave up or did not even begin. We have been advised to accumulate 30 minutes of any exercise that is aerobic throughout the day. The experts are even suggesting that doing 10 minutes of exercise per day can be of great benefit. This is good news because it is encouraging to know that every little bit helps. But it could also mean that we're so badly out of shape as a nation, that even the slightest movement is an improvement. Sort of like a junk food junkie drinking one less Coke a day, you might say.

However, for the absolute best results, it is strongly recommended that you aim to do no less than 30-45 minutes during each session. The time spent on the aerobic activity excludes the warm-up and the cool-down. After just 20 minutes, your fat releasing enzymes have kicked in and are releasing fat which is being burned for up to 36 hours after aerobic exercise.

This is quite easy to do if you have decided that you are going to take up walking or jogging, because you leave the front door and don't return for the next 45 minutes. However, in the gym, spending 45 minutes on one piece of cardiovascular equipment can become quite mundane. What I recommend in this situation is to move around different machines. For example, I will spend 10 minutes on the treadmill, then five minutes on the rowing machine, then another 10 minutes on the Stairmaster, and finish up with 10 minutes on the bike. Each time I will mix it around by doing more time on some than others and changing the order around as well. It never seems to get boring!

If you find that occasionally there are days that you simply cannot fit 30-45 minutes at a time, research shows that breaking the aerobic section up into two sessions is just as beneficial. Therefore, in this situation, you could squeeze 15 minutes on the stairmaster first thing in the morning and hopefully be able to do a power walk at lunchtime. Obviously, you could use any other preferred aerobic activity to complete the two sections.

Exercise frequency:

How quickly do you want to see changes in your body shape? The answer will determine your frequency. I've seen a great success rate with a frequency of 3-5 times per week. Research shows that the difference between exercising aerobically twice a week or three times a week is quite significant. Working out three times a week may sound like a lot at first, but if you think about it realistically, it is only less than two hours a week!

It is strongly recommended that you don't put your aerobic exercise off to the last minute, which is why it is not a bad idea to try and fit it in first thing in the morning. That way, you have done it and you can spare yourself the excuses later. Many of us are not morning people, I do realize. Actually, there is no evidence to suggest that exercising in the morning is more beneficial than at any other time of the day, regardless of what certain popular fitness trainers have been saying to us.

When I was in London, I recall being quite surprised one evening to see one of my friend's husband running past the Natural History Museum at 10:00 p.m.! That was "his" time. He went on to complete several marathons. Exercising first thing in the morning has the positive advantage of making you feel energized for the whole day. Somehow, sitting down to breakfast after you have been out exercising for an hour seems so well earned!

Exercise intensity:

How long you exercise and how often you exercise are equally important, but not as important as intensity. If you are not working-out at the right intensity, you are unlikely to see dramatic results and will probably end up feeling frustrated. This is something I see very often in the gym—the same faces every day and unfortunately, the same bodies. No change. This is because they do not make the effort to put a little more effort into their intensity. They don't want to perspire too much as it might ruin their hair. Or, they end up chatting endlessly to the person on the treadmill next to them.

Intensity has been much the topic of debate in the past few years. The target Heart Rate Chart was formerly used to prescribe aerobic exercise within a target zone of 60-90 percent of age-predicted maximum heart rate (Age-PMHR). Now we have a newly developed Heart Rate Guide showing that even small increases above resting heart rate may be beneficial to health, while greater increases can provide both health and fitness benefits. Since most of the population is chronically inactive, the reasoning is *better something than nothing!*

When researchers compared high-intensity exercise with endurance training, they found the more vigorous work out produced greater fat loss. They concluded that vigorous exercise (about 70 percent of maximum heart rate) for 45-60 minutes caused an increase in fat-burning enzymes, a greater rise in resting metabolic rate and therefore greater weight loss in the long run. For maximizing "fat burning," the key is to work as long as possible at as high an intensity as possible in order to maximize calorie burning. This can be implemented as you get fitter. In other words, you can work harder for longer periods of time.

Overall:
Select one or more aerobic activities of your choice.
Exercise aerobically 3-5 times per week.
Work out for a minimum of 30-45 minutes each session.
Work out at a moderate intensity in the beginning.
As you become more fit, increase your intensity.
Vary your workouts often and cross train.

Now, let's undo a little myth that seems to have been blown out of all proportion in the health clubs of America. Suddenly, everyone started talking about slowing down to burn more fat...and slowing down they were! There were even clubs advertising "fat burning classes." I think that some are still doing it. The theory is that if you kept the intensity down, the primary fuel utilized would be fat, and if you allowed the intensity to go up too high, then you were not burning fat but rather carbohy-drates as fuel. It is true that you burn a higher percentage of fat calories during low-intensity exercise. The primary fuel we burn all day long is fat. So naturally, when you increase your intensi-ty even slightly, the fat fuel will burn up quicker.

However, as exercise intensity increases, so does the overall rate at which all calories are burned—whether they are carbohydrates or fats. Therefore, the total percentage of calories used is greater. This means the total amount of fat burned is also higher. But, if you are not fit, it is advisable to start out at a lower intensity. This will stimulate the fat cells to start releasing fat. If you try and work at an intensity that is too high to begin with and your body is not at that level of fitness, the results will be discouraging. The systems are not adapted to this training, which would be anaerobic and force the body to burn a higher percentage of carbohydrates and not fat.

While aerobic exercise will accomplish cardiorespiratory fitness, let's take a closer look at strength training and its bene-fits. As scientists are now battling the final enemy—human aging, once considered an inevitable cause of muscle weakness, bone loss, sluggish metabolism, and a slow but sure loss of func-tion, they have concluded that the weapon of choice is strength training. You certainly don't have to decline with age.

You can actually control and even reverse signs of aging through weight-bearing exercise. After all, for every 72 hours you are idle, you can lose up to five percent of your muscle strength, depending upon your level of fitness. In fact, if you are not participating in any weight-bearing activity, you are losing strength so gradually that you probably haven't noticed. But you will.

Eighteen or 80, today's men and women who understand that good health, high energy and stamina equate with youth, have turned to strength training in a disciplined and sensible way. This also known as resistance training, which can be achieved through the use of calisthenics, weight machines and systems, and free weights. Those who actively weight train benefit from increased fat-free mass, increased bone density, improved functional strength, improved posture, and muscle balance. A strength training study at Boston's Tuft's University showed that those who weight train are onto one of the smartest routines to longevity.

You can actually control and even reverse signs of aging through weight-bearing exercise.

The researchers believe that strength training can help prevent and even reverse some of the physical effects of aging. Strength training can control all metabolic dysfunction, strength loss, and fat gain. Furthermore, strength training may be vital to creating just the right combination of muscle, bone, and fat in your body. The Tufts study examined the impact of walking and calcium supplementation on bone mass, for example. They found that both strengthen the skeleton, but at two different places: calcium boosting bone at the thigh bone, and exercise preventing bone loss at the spine. "When a woman loses 20 or 30 pounds, she loses both muscle and bone, which may compromise her health," says Dr. Miriam Nelson, the study leader. "Adding strength training to the weight-loss program can prevent dangerous muscle and bone loss."

A group of obese women were put on a calorie-restricted diet in a University of Michigan study, and either weight trained or didn't do much exercise at all. They all lost about the same amount of weight. But the sedentary women lost two pounds of lean muscle mass while the strength-training group gained a pound of muscle and lost a greater percentage of fat.

At the age of 20, the average woman has 23 percent body fat and the average man has 18 percent. At age 35, the women are at 30 percent and the men at 20 percent. At age 60, a woman's body fat is at 44 percent and a man's is at 38 percent. Frankly, the less muscle you have, the lower your metabolism— and the easier it is to gain weight.

Contrary to what many of us believe, aerobic exercise doesn't stop this muscle-to-fat progression. Studies indicate that endurance-sport enthusiasts lose large amounts of muscle mass and strength by their 60s, even if aerobically fit. The strength-trained, however, maintain muscle size and strength well into their 70s. When Danish researchers studied 70-year-old men who swam, ran or lifted weights regularly, they concluded that the swimmers and runners had lost as much as sedentary 70-year-olds, while the weight lifters had muscle strength and com-position comparable to 28-year-olds.

Today, most women who exercise attend aerobic classes or they jog, and they consider themselves fit as a result. But take a realistic look at them. The vast majority rarely utilize the weight room. Aerobics participants define their fitness regimen only in terms of cardiovascular training, which obviously has its value as discussed previously.

Falsely, they actually think they are getting stronger in their low-impact, step, funk, and high-low classes. Realistically, most of them cannot do half a dozen consecutive push-ups and rarely is there a noted change in their body composition or posture. However, simple exercises such as leg lifts, sit-ups, and knee extensions have shown extraordinary results. One of the most valuable outcomes of the exercise program followed at Tufts University was a gain in muscle mass as well as muscle strength. Weight-bearing or resistance exercises certainly can have a profoundly positive impact on the quality of our lives, regardless of age.

The researchers report increases in the strength of the muscles in the women's legs, backs, abdomens, and buttocks average from an astonishing 35-76 percent. The extra muscle power, in turn, made it easier to become more active, to engage in activities that previously they simply lacked the energy to perform. They really became more youthful, noted the researchers. After one year of strength training, they emerged physiologically younger by 15-20 years than when they began. Even their psychological profiles were much more youthful.

Until recently, strength training has been possibly the most misunderstood and under-rated of all athletic and fitness activities.

Until recently, strength training has been possibly the most misunderstood and under-rated of all athletic and fitness activities. As a result, too many of us have passed it up. But even a minimal strength training regimen increases stamina, develops muscle tone and strength, improves athletic performance, and various other benefits.

Those who fear they may become bulky with weight training need not worry. Strength training is not the same as bodybuilding. You will achieve muscle tone, definition and strength, not bulk or size. You will not become a topographical marvel like Arnold Schwarzenegger. Strength for health and longevity is as different from body building as recreational jogging is from running in the Olympics.

Understanding how our muscles work underscores how important strength training can be. The body's movements rely on the condition of the more than 600 skeletal muscles comprising it. Skeletal muscles are those that are attached to the bones by tendons. These muscles are collections of tiny fibers consistent of two types of cells, fast-twitch and slow-twitch, that contract and relax when directed by nerve impulses from the brain. Fast-twitch cells react quickly and powerfully, allowing us to move rapidly for short periods of time and to exert maximal strength output.

However, as glycogen is used up, muscle fatigue sets in. Slow-twitch cells metabolize oxygen directly from the blood and are constantly supplied with energy. They can sustain action over long periods of time and are also responsible for static activities like standing and maintaining posture. The major muscle groups contain different ratios of both cells depending on their function. A well-conditioned muscle cell is able to contract to about half of its resting length and can support more than

1,000 times its own weight—but this ability diminishes with age beginning in the late 30s and by the age of 65 can be reduced by between 20-40 percent. A balanced strength regimen can help keep your losses to a minimum.

It is interesting to know that the strength-trainers in the Tuft's study didn't actually shed any pounds because as they burned off body fat, they added to the weight of their muscle. But the shift in the proportion of fat to lean muscle tissue gave them a trimmer look. It is not unusual to lose two dress sizes and not a single pound of weight from strength training.

Strength training by itself leads to more calories spent. Researchers point out that it is not that the exercises on their own that are big calorie burners, it's that they increase the calories burned when you are NOT exercising. That is because the muscles they build require extra calories to "service" or maintain them. Another way of putting it is that strength training activates the rate in which the body burns calories to sustain itself while you are resting. Technically, it is known as the Resting Metabolic Rate (RMR) and is defined as the pace at which calories are burned at rest. This is closely linked to the amount of muscle in your body. The loss of muscle

The greater your strength, the less likely you are to become fatigued and feel tired and sluggish—both physically and mentally.

slows down your RMR, thus fewer calories are burned. Therefore, with loss of muscle, your chance for long-term weight loss success is low. RMR accounts for 60-75 percent of your daily energy expenditure. The key to successful long-term weight loss is to understand the importance of increasing the amount of muscle in your body. Even a modest increase in your RMR can favorably influence your body composition. As RMR goes up, more calories will be burned during all activities, including sitting, lying down, and sleeping. Every pound of muscle added to the body burns about 35 extra calories per day, or about 3-4 pounds of fat every year.

Besides burning extra calories and becoming more active in their daily lives, the Tufts subjects increased their bone density and as a result put off osteoporosis. After a single year of strength training, the women increased the bone mass in their hips and lower spines by an average of one percent, the researchers reported.

A similar group of sedentary women, on the other hand, lost some 2.5 percent density in their hip bones and spines. Accumulated over the years, the researchers say that such differences could make the non-exercisers more than two and a half times as likely as the exercisers to suffer a debilitating fracture. They further noted that as a result of strength training, the risk of developing diabetes and high cholesterol are decreased. Another key finding by Tufts is that the strength trainers improved their balance by 14 percent, as opposed to a 9 percent decline in balance in the sedentary women.

Increasingly studies show that we lose muscle mainly because we use it less as we age. Strength training can help stave off the body composition changes that occur primarily between the ages of 35 and 55. This is the time to pay attention to prevention because once you are up in years, body composition is stable and body fat is quite high.

It's never too late to begin strength training, though. When the U.S. Department of Agriculture Research Center on Aging at Tufts University studied a group of 90-year-old men and women, they found that the seniors increased their strength by an average of 174 percent after just eight weeks of twice-weekly work-outs on weight machines. In another study, Tufts put a group of 87-96 year olds on a strength training program to discover that every single subject had increased his/her strength by 300-400 percent. Researchers have concluded that even if you strength train just once a week for at least 10 weeks, at a minimum of two or three times per week, you will maintain and even improve your function.

Scientists claim that all the time you need to give to strength training is 45 minutes twice a week and you will get back 15 to 20 years of youthfulness. If you are now in your 20s, 30s, or 40s, your youth will simply become more vital and vigorous.

Indeed, a quiet transformation has been sweeping the world of anti-aging seekers and it's all about getting stronger and feeling younger. It all makes sense.

Exercise causes the biggest jump in life expectancy for people who go from doing nothing to being even moderately active.

The greater your strength, the less likely you are to become fatigued and feel tired and sluggish—both physically and mentally. The stronger you are, the more active and challenging you are. After all, is anything associated more with youth than energy?

The fittest people are the most active and hence, the most interested and interesting. Exercise causes the biggest jump in life expectancy for people who go from doing nothing to being even moderately active. In fact, exercise wields such an enormously powerful effect that if you have high blood pressure, for example, and you exercise, you will have a greater life expectancy than if you have normal blood pressure and you don't exercise.

What all this shows is that an increase in weakness and frailty as we age is not a given. Like most things in life, here too, you have a choice. We do not have to accept the grim stereotype of aging as an unalterable process of decline and loss. The earlier in life you start strength training, the better off you'll be by the time you hit the seventh, eighth, and ninth decade of life.

A suggested meal plan to help increase your endurance, strength, and flexibility.

<u>On rising:</u>
Drink a glass of water with a rounded teaspoon of acidophilus. Half an hour later: Drink one-ounce of wheatgrass* juice. Drink a glass of fresh carrot juice with bee pollen and propolis.

<u>Breakfast:</u>
Whole grain toast and plain yogurt, or multigrain hot cereal and goat's milk, or grilled vegetables and eggs or tofu. Hot cup of green tea.
Supplements: vitamin C, vitamin E, vitamins B-complex, a multi vitamin/mineral.

<u>Mid-morning:</u>
Hot potassium broth or crunchy vegetables of your choice. Hawthorn berry extract in small amount of room temperature water.

<u>Lunch:</u>
Whole grains in any form, nuts and/or beans; or raw dairy products or tofu, and other soy foods of your choice with vegetables that are grilled, steamed, or fresh. A hot cup of green tea with lemongrass.**

---

* *Wheatgrass has enormous curative powers for numerous degenerative "incurable" diseases when taken as a fresh liquid. It is arguably the best "preventive" tonic from nature. Fifteen pounds of fresh wheat grass is equal in nutritional value to 350 pounds of the choicest vegetables. In tablet or powder form it provides highly concentrated food for those who need more dietary greens and roughage.*

** *Lemongrass is used for its astringent and tonic properties. It works well in combination with green tea which combats fatigue and lowers the risk of esophageal, stomach, colon, and skin cancer and delays the onset of arteriosclerosis.*

Supplements: vitamin C, vitamin E, vitamins B-complex, a multi vitamin/mineral, and Kyolic garlic.

Mid-afternoon:
Fresh fruit in season. Echinacea and ginkgo extracts. Alfalfa tablets.

Dinner:
Brown rice or whole grain breads and seafood or chicken or occasional organic beef with steamed vegetables and/or a fresh green salad with olive oil, fresh lemon, garlic, and herbs of your choice. A hot cup of chamomile*** tea.
Supplements: vitamin C and Kyolic garlic.

Bedtime:
A hot potassium broth and a glass of room temperature spring water with phyllium husks or a mild senna tea.

***

*** *Chamomile is an anti-inflammatory, appetite stimulant, digestive aid, diuretic, nerve tonic, and sleep aid. It helps colitis, diverticulosis, fever, headaches, and pain. Chamomile is a traditional remedy for stress and anxiety, indigestion, and insomnia.*

CHAPTER 12
HOW TO MAINTAIN YOUR BODY TRANSFORMATION

When we mistreat the machine that we live in, body transformation becomes vital. The human machine is unique and very special in that it carries all the equipment we require to function. This includes its own drug factory, energy processing station, and computer/information system.

For all of these systems and others to function optimally, the machine needs fuel and components that help in creating the peptides, cells and channels of information to complete their jobs. If those items are missing, then the system will begin to break down and the machine starts having problems like cancer, Alzheimer's, skin problems, and yes, even old age. The body machine is for our use so that we may function in this world and interact with each other. In many ways, the body is but a physical, mental, and spiritual computer.

To keep the system functioning correctly we must not ignore the very specific fuel that it must have. In today's world it is very difficult to eat the right healthy foods. Most everything we eat is processed and those processes eliminate many of the important items as we have discussed in the previous chapters.

High energy foods like sugar-filled products and other man-made synthetic products can be very dangerous in that they cause the body to function at a much faster rate than what it is designed or trained for. An example can be found in how the old steam engine would work. The coal process would create high energy, but in short bursts. It had its use, but the remnants from the coal would create blockages that could become explosive if not regularly cleaned out. Wood, on the other hand, would not clog the system as badly and would last longer in the energy consumption. People need the same training in this process; then, many of the problems we encounter with diseases and premature aging would be greatly decreased or eliminated.

On more than one occasion during the writing of this book, my editors would review the dietary recommendations and say, "Julie, lighten up!" Often, we really do resist any degree of change in our lives, even when it becomes life threatening. Let's take a look at cancer victims. Of those who survive cancer, nearly 80 percent of them get the disease again within five years. Why? Because they can beat the disease, but usually not the lifestyle that led to it in the first place; therefore, they get the

> **Of those who survive cancer, nearly 80% of them get the disease again within five years. Why? Because they can beat the disease, but usually not the lifestyle that led to it in the first place; therefore, they get the illness again.**

illness again. The same can be said for heart disease, the #1 killer of men and women.

Change may not be easily welcomed, but most of us know that those who do not evolve perish. Evolution is not possible without wellness and optimal health is by no means a given. Modern medicine defines health as the absence of disease. If it were only that simple! If one doesn't suffer from diabetes or cancer or heart disease, then by definition, one is healthy. This is a lie. A healthy individual is in a state of high resistance to illness and one who thrives physically, emotionally, mentally, and spiritually.

Natural health possesses a powerful immune system. Artificial health is a modern definition. People reach old age, but only with the reliance on drugs and invasive, intrusive medical intervention. This is a dependency state. It is an inferior state of health and we recognize this truth intuitively. Much of our dissatisfaction with doctors today is that they don't teach us about healthy living.

Yet, it is an increasingly unhealthy lifestyle that sends us marching to doctor's offices. The number one reason for doctors' visits is fatigue—from mild to severe. This low energy state is debilitating to every single aspect of a person's life. After all, health depends upon the required release of energy found in the food we eat. This energy has to be released continuously and efficiently in every bodily cell in order to function optimally. A variety of vitamins, minerals, trace minerals, and other substances have to be available at the required dosages for maximal energy production. An imbalance of any kind in this fuel system will sap your energy, resulting in fatigue and feelings of exhaustion.

> Only a true commitment to health, a properly digested and monitored diet in combination with adequate exercise, as well as other integrated therapies, will bring a person to a state of natural good health.

Whether you call it fatigue, exhaustion or burnout, often it is blamed on stress. During my own energy crisis, every single doctor would ask immediately, "Julie, are you under stress?" To which I'd reply, "Doctor, are you under stress?" We are ALL under stress, but don't make that issue a sweeping generality and ignore other serious and potentially threatening health concerns. Chronic fatigue is a breakdown of the energy systems of the body that can actually cause depression, withdrawal or feelings of hopelessness. Fatigue is a physical condition that can be reversed by rebuilding body chemistry. Your attitude can and usually does contribute to your level of physical exhaustion and emotional stress, but it's not ALL in your head.

Further, we assume that burned-out people just mope around all the time. In reality, they usually have full-time jobs, raise families, and may even present the illusion of good health. But don't be fooled. Those folks are tired, irritable, and require stimulants to keep going—coffee, colas, high sugar content foods, alcohol, antidepressants, pain killers, sleeping pills, and the like. Some engage in manic exercise, falsely assuming that a killer work out will boost their energy level. A temporary time-out does not resolve chronic fatigue either. Only a true commitment to health, a properly digested and monitored diet in combination with adequate exercise, as well as other integrated therapies, will bring a person to a state of natural good health.

Those of us who have experienced devastating health crises personally and/or among our family and friends, realize all too well that there is only prevention and that a healthy lifestyle absolutely must be our number one priority. We're not talking about an obsessive preoccupation but an arsenal of knowledge accompanied by disciplined planning and preparation. Otherwise, distractions will inevitably arise throughout the day and you will find yourself forced into unhealthy choices with undesirable consequences.

If we can look for a positive angle to this national epidemic of chronic exhaustion and obesity, it is that we are led to examine our lifestyle. But just taking a closer look isn't enough. You must take action and rebuild your body chemistry to correct the imbalances that caused your fatigue and weight issues in the first place.

In *Body Transformation*, I encourage you to give up modern *foods* and return to foods that nature gave us in abundance to thrive. Whole grains have been available to man for thousands of years. White bread is a very *new food*—bleached white for good looks and fluffiness. It is "enriched" for our health as some 40 nutrients are taken out so the white waste matter can then be enriched with FOUR nutrients—not by choice mind you, but by law! This is because white bread was found to be dangerously deficient in vital nutrients. Unfortunately, white bread isn't the only culprit, as we discussed. I think that all those cute, sugary, colorful cold cereals make great packing material. Colas are very effective for cleaning the terminals on your car battery. Margarine makes a fine bicycle grease. However, don't eat it!

Throughout this book, I insist on organic foods. Until modern times, this was the ONLY method of growing food. Do you want to eat foods laced with chemicals so deadly that they have decimated entire animal species? It is now known that pesticides, for instance, have the same gene-altering effects as atomic radiation.

In our 50 states, more than 2,000,000,000 pounds of herbicides, fungicides, and pesticides are routinely sprayed on the crops that we eat. The harm this does to us is not news. President Kennedy's science advisor, Dr. Jerome Weisner, testified before Congress: "Using agricultural pesticides is more dangerous than atomic fallout!"

These days, even the American Cancer Society, famous for their silent stance about environmental and nutritional causes of cancer, stated that up to 80 percent of cancers might be environmentally caused as we are "losing the war on cancer."

In general, we are told that we are living better and longer than ever, but this is just not so. Today, Americans rank 21st in life expectancy. Much of this is attributed to a fast food diet and a fast-paced lifestyle. It is now recognized that energies are present within each food that affects our physical and mental functioning. Let's look at our most abused *food* substance once again—sugar. The Journal of Biosocial Research reported that the average person eats about 150 pounds of sugar each year. Juvenile delinquents in custody eat about 300 pounds of sugar a year. When this sugar intake was significantly reduced, junk food was reduced, and fruits and vegetables were increased, there was a 48 percent decrease in antisocial behavior of all types. This was true for all ages and races—at no cost to the taxpayer.

"Conscious eating" must once again become the norm for all society to achieve physical, mental, and spiritual optimal health. Never before have we possessed so much knowledge, had such an abundance and variety of food and yet suffered such devastating consequences because of poor choice. Thus, *Body Transformation* is not a fad, but a *necessity*.

In several weeks time, you will have made tremendous strides. As Socrates once said, "There is only one good—knowledge, and one evil—ignorance." As you grow in knowledge, patience, and discipline, and allow nature to do the healing and rebuilding, you will experience a physical and mental transformation that will serve you for as long as you live. Do not fear that if you have slipped off the program or cut an occasional corner that it's all out the window. Remember, as you reach for the stars and only get as far as the moon, you will be much farther along than most.

As your body detoxifies and becomes pure and vibrant, you will be able to introduce "fun" foods into your diet, in moderation, and usually not suffer consequences. In fact, as your eating habits become very healthy and your body renews itself, you will be able to decrease the amounts of supplements you take as well as the thought process that goes into planning and making food choices. It will become second nature.

My personal weakness is chocolate and two mischievous fellows named Ben & Jerry. I have been blessed with numerous sweet teeth. If I could live on a chocolate diet, I would. I tried. Believe me, I tried. As I have gotten my body into a very pure state at this time, I allow myself sweets on holidays and birthdays. This resolution has often led me to scour the calendar for any saints and presidents that are being honored.

The body transformation way of life represents the collective wisdom of thousands of health seekers from Biblical times to modern science.

However, the adverse effects that follow such an indulgence soon make themselves known and I regret having given into my craving almost immediately. It reminds me that healthy food choices are my real reward. If, on occasion, I choose to go completely mad and devour everything made of chocolate in my orbit, I do it at a time when I can afford to mope, agonize, and suffer in general so not to allow the ill effects to interfere with my responsibility to work and the people around me. For instance, after being hit in the head with a golf ball while taking a stroll on Christmas morning, I was forced into a virtually complete state of inactivity. At the same time, I went on a "brain food" diet, increasing omega-3 oil-rich foods, certain proteins, and vegetables. I also ate every two hours to keep the energy steady. Of course, it being the holiday season, the pumpkin pies and cheesecakes had my name all over them. Further, I couldn't insult all the well wishers who sent me chocolates and baskets of goodies! A little indulgence here and there led not only to several extra pounds on the scale, but to bouts of moodiness, depression, and disturbed sleep. Only then do I once again realize that it's far better to stay healthy then it is to go through yet another "reversal" process.

You too, in due course, will intuitively know what works best for you and how to stick with the program. As Thomas Edison once said, "The doctor of the future will give no medicine but will interest his patients in the care of the human frame, in proper diet, and in the cause and prevention of disease." The light of applied understanding always weakens our physical and mental malfunctions.

The body transformation way of life represents the collective wisdom of thousands of health seekers from Biblical times to modern science. The advice offered in this book is based on science as well as ancient wisdom and has been shown to work. We should aim to live a natural and not a drug-based life. I have experienced healing personally and have likewise witnessed the transformation of countless others.

The body transformation way of life is very cost-effective in the long run as well. The focus is on physical and mental well being. It emphasizes prevention. It looks at the cause and not just the symptoms. You may be asking yourself, if the body transformation way of eating, supplementing, and working-out is really sound, then why hasn't your doctor steered you in a similar direction? The answer is very simple. Your doctor is an expert on disease, not health. Ironically, the health care industry is in the business of illness rather than well being. You wouldn't ask your doctor about healthy eating and exercise any more than you'd ask him to repair your car or install your satellite dish. Unless he had taken it up as a personal interest, it's just out of his realm of expertise. Even when good research is put before the doctors, they are oddly resistant. Remember, if all you're trained to use is a hammer, the whole world looks like a nail.

It takes time and diligence for new ideas to take hold and become the norm. During the early 1800s in Vienna, for example, a doctor had the audacity to suggest to his fellow physicians that they wash their hands after they finished working on cadavers, rather than using their unwashed hands to deliver babies, so to avoid infecting the women and their children. However, his colleagues ridiculed him. It took them 30 years to catch on and wash their hands. Imagine how many babies died because the doctors thought they knew it all?

Body transformation began for me when my own body and thus life, came into jeopardy. Although I possessed the will, fierce determination, diligence, and a good deal of time, money, and resources to transform myself as needed, I realized that such options are not available to most people. This is why I wrote this book and why so many wonderful people contributed to its creation and endorsement. I am merely the messenger and not the creator. At the end of the day, the good news is that most everything that happens to us is reversible—*if we apply ourselves.*

Eating and physical activity are two of the greatest joys in life. Food and exercise are a pleasure, an absolute necessity and not a punishment. By learning how healthy choices affect your body and mind, you will master the secret to success in any area of your life. What the first of the Sibyls at Delphi, Herophile, stated in 300 B.C. is still true: "When health is absent, wisdom cannot reveal itself, art cannot become manifest, strength cannot be exerted. Wealth is useless, and reason is powerless." As you continue with the body transformation way of life, you will increasingly experience a state of health and youthfulness that you didn't think possible. You will actually experience a state of agelessness as your chronological age stand still and your pathological age improves. As you attain a toxic-free body, you will reach the heights of physical, mental, and spiritual evolution. This will add many youthful, active, and joyous years to your life.

*   *   *

GLOSSARY

Acidophilus A nutritional supplement containing bacteria with a symbiotic, or mutually beneficial, relationship with the human stomach. It helps break down complex food molecules and inhibits the growth of harmful bacteria. It is especially useful for people with bacterial or yeast infections, or digestive problems, as well as those taking antibiotics. Products of this type are generally referred to as probiotics.

Allergy An immune malfunction whereby a person's body is hyposensitized to react immunologically to typically nonimmunogenic substances. When a person is hyposensitized, these substances are known as allergens. An allergic response to a substance may vary from a runny nose to life-threatening anaphylactic shock and death.

Aloe Vera juice The aloe vera plant consists of a large variety of amino acids, enzymes, vitamins, and minerals. It comes closer than any other known plant to the duplication of life's essential substances in the biochemistry of the human body. Aloe vera has natural healing and detoxifying powers and works gently within the intestinal tract to help break down impacted food residues and thoroughly cleanse the bowel. It can help ease constipation and prevent continuing diarrhea, setting a regularity to the bowel. Further, aloe vera speeds up cell growth, is a stimulant to the immune system, a powerful anti-inflammatory, and an analgesic. Aloe vera contains a large number of mucopolysaccharides (basic sugars) that are found in every cell in the body. Aloe also contains large numbers of nutrients including vitamins E, C, B1, B2, B3, and B6 as well as iron, manganese, calcium, and zinc. Seven essential amino acids are also found in aloe vera.

Amino acid Any of 22 nitrogen-containing organic acids from which proteins are made.

Anemia A deficiency of red blood cells and/or hemoglobin. This results in a reduced ability of blood to transfer oxygen to the tissues. Hemoglobin (the oxygen-carrying protein in the red blood cells) has to be present to ensure adequate oxygenation of all body tissues and organs.

Anorexia A decreased sensation of appetite. While the term in non-scientific publications is often used interchangeably with one of its subtypes, anorexia nervosa, there are many possible causes for the decreased appetite, some of which may be harmless while others pose significant risk to the person.

Antidepressant A medication designed to treat or alleviate the symptoms of clinical depression. Some antidepressants, notably the tricyclics, are commonly used off-label in the treatment of neuropathic pain, whether or not the patient is depressed. Many antidepressants are also used for the treatment of anxiety disorders.

Antioxidant A chemical that prevents the oxidation of other chemicals. In biological systems, the normal processes of oxidation produce highly reactive free radicals. These can readily react with and damage other molecules. In some cases, the body uses this to fight infection. In other cases, the damage may be the body's own cells. The presence of extremely easily oxidizable compounds in the system can "mop up" free radicals before they damage other essential molecules. Virtually all studies of mammals have concluded that a restricted calorie diet extends the lifespan of mammals by as much as 100%. This remarkable finding suggests that food is actually more damaging than smoking, which takes on average 25% of a person's lifespan. As food produces free radicals (oxidants) when metabolized, antioxidant-rich diets are thought to stave off the effects of aging significantly better than antioxidant-poor diets.

Astragalus An herb that's a powerful immunomodulator.

Bioflavanoids The pigments occurring in plants responsible for the colors of fruits and flowers. One of the main activities of bioflavanoids is to scavenge compounds called free radicals, which damage cell membranes. Free radical damage is involved in aging, cancer, and damage to blood vessels that permits the development of atherosclerosis. Bioflavanoids also decrease cholesterol levels in the blood as well as the oxidation of cholesterol, decreasing the chance of plaque formation.

Blood pressure The pressure exerted by the blood on the walls of the blood vessels. Typical values for the arterial blood pressure of a resting, healthy adult are approximately 120/80. Blood pressure is not static, but undergoes natural variations from one heartbeat to another or throughout the day; it also changes in response to stress, nutritional factors, drugs or disease.

Body mass index (BMI) A calculated number based on height and weight used to compare and analyze the health effects of weight on human bodies of all heights. BMI is a common means of measuring high weights and obesity in humans.

Bulimia An eating disorder. It is a psychological condition in which the subject engages in recurrent binge eating followed by intentionally doing one or more of the following in order to compensate for the intake of the food and prevent weight gain: vomiting; inappropriate use of laxatives, enemas, diuretics and other medication, excessive exercising, and fasting.

Carbohydrates Chemical compounds that contain oxygen, hydrogen, and carbon atoms. Certain carbohydrates are an important storage and transport form of energy in most organisms, including plants and animals. Carbohydrates are classified by the number of sugar units into monosaccharides (such as glucose), disaccharides (such as saccharose), oligosaccharides, and polysaccharides (such as starch, glycogen, and cellulose).

Cardiovascular disease Diseases affecting the heart or blood vessels, which include: atherosclerosis, coronary artery disease, heart valve disease, stroke, arrhythmia, heart failure, hypertension, orthostatic hypotension, shock, endocarditis, diseases of the aorta and its branches, disorders of the peripheral vascular system, and congenital heart disease.

Cell (biology) The structural and functional unit of all living organisms. Cells are sometimes called the "building blocks of life." A bacterium is a single-cell organism but a human being is estimated to have some 100,000 billion cells. All vital functions of an organism occur within cells. Cells contain the hereditary information necessary for regulating cell functions; they transmit information to the next generation of cells.

Cesium 137 A rare and dangerous radioactive isotope of cesium. Cesium 137 is produced from the detonation of nuclear weapons and is produced in nuclear power plants, most notably from the 1986 Chernobyl meltdown.

Chamomile tea Made from chamomile flowers, it helps to relax tense muscles, reduce stress, anxiety, and exhaustion. It is also used to balance acidity and eases indigestion and gastritis. Chamomile is also an anti-inflammatory and helps with eczema.

Chaparral tea Though technically an herb, the leaves and twigs of this evergreen desert shrub are used to make tea. The active ingredient of chaparral is a potent antioxidant. Chaparral tea is a well-known and old Indian remedy that has been used for a wide variety of ailments, including arthritis, cancer, venereal disease, bowel cramps, rheumatism, and colds. It is said to possess analgesic, expectorant, emetic, diuretic, and anti-inflammatory properties.

Chlorella A collective name for a single-celled algae. Chlorella contains chlorophyll and is about 45% protein, 20% fat, 20% sugar, and 15% various vitamins and minerals.

Chlorophyll A green photosynthetic pigment found in plants, algae, and cyanobacteria.

Cholesterol A crystalline substance that is soluble in fats and produced by all vertebrates. It is a necessary constituent of cell membranes, and facilitates the transport and absorption of fatty acids. Excess cholesterol, however, is a potential threat to health.

Cobalt-60 A radioactive isotope of the element cobalt. One gram of cobalt-60 contains approximately 50 curies. Held at close range, this amount of cobalt-60 would irradiate a person with approximately 0.g gray of ionizing radiation per minute. A full body dose of approximately 3-4 sieverts will kill 50% of the population in 30 days, and could be accumulated in just a few minutes of exposure to a gram of cobalt-60. Cobalt-60 has four main uses: as a tracer for cobalt in chemical reactors; sterilization of medical equipment; as a radioactive source for food irradiation; and as a radioactive source for laboratory use

Coenzyme A molecule that works with an enzyme to enable the enzyme to perform its function in the body. Coenzymes are necessary in the utilization of vitamins and minerals.

Cold-pressed A term used to describe food oils that are extracted without the use of heat in order to preserve nutrients and flavor.

Complex carbohydrates A type of carbohydrate that, owing to its chemical structure, releases its sugar into the body relatively slowly and also provides fiber. The carbohydrates in starches and fiber are complex carbohydrates. Also called polysaccharides.

Depression An everyday term used for a sad or low mood or the loss of pleasure, but not clustered with other symptoms of clinical depression or a sustained change in brain chemistry. Clinical depression is a medically-defined state of mind identified by clusters of symptoms such as markedly-decreased motivation, interest, libido, activity, sense of pleasure, ability to sleep, etc.

Detoxification The process of reducing the building up of various poisonous substances in the body.

DHEA Dehydroepiandrosterone (DHEA) is a natural steroid hormone produced from cholesterol by the adrenal glands found atop the kidneys in the human body. DHEA is also produced in the gonads, adipose tissue, and the brain. DHEA is structurally similar to, and is a precursor of, androstenedione, testosterone, and estrogen. It is the most abundant hormone in the body.

Diabetes mellitus A medical disorder characterized by varying or persistent hyperglycemia (high blood sugar), especially after eating. All types of diabetes mellitus share similar symptoms and complications at advanced stages. Hyperglycemia itself can lead to dehydration and ketoacidosis. Longer-term complications include cardiovascular disease (double risk); chronic renal failure (the main cause for dialysis); retinal damage that can lead to blindness; nerve damage which can lead to erectile dysfunction (impotence); gangrene with risk of amputation of toes, feet, and even legs. The more serious complications are more common in people who have a difficult time controlling their blood sugars with medications or if the disease is left untreated.

Digestion The process whereby a biological entity processes a substance in order to chemically convert the substance into nutrients. Digestion occurs at the cellular and sub-cellular levels. Digestion begins in the mouth where food is chewed with the teeth. The process stimulates exocrine glands in the mouth to release digestive enzymes such as salivary amylase, which aid in the breakdown of food, particularly carbohydrates. Chewing also causes the release of saliva, which helps condense food into a bolus that can be easily passed through the esophagus to the stomach. In the stomach, food is churned and thoroughly mixed with acid and other digestive enzymes with digestive fluid to further decompose it chemically. As the acidic level changes in the stomach and later parts of the digestive tract, more enzymes are activated or deactivated to extract and process various nutrients. After being processed in the stomach, food is passed to the small intestine. It is pushed through the small intestine via a process called peristalsis, a squeezing action, before it passes through the sphincter where it is further mixed with secretions such as bile, which helps aid in fat digestion, and the enzymes maltase, lactase, and sucrase, to process sugars. Most nutrient absorption takes place in the small intestine, after which food is passed to the large intestine. Blood which has absorbed nutrients passes through the liver for filtering, removal of toxins, and help in processing of nutrients. In the large intestine, water is reabsorbed and leftover waste is excreted by defecation.

Echinacea Today, the Echinacea herb is primarily used to reduce the symptoms and duration of the common cold and flu and to alleviate the symptoms associated with them, such as sore throat, cough, and fever. It also helps boost the activity of the immune system to help the body fight infections. The

University of Maryland reports that the latest animal studies suggest that Echinacea controls active substances that enhance the activity of the immune system, relieve pain, reduce inflammation, and have hormonal, antiviral, and antioxidant effects.

Elderflower tea Elder has certain therapeutic properties and the reported benefits of using it internally in the form of an herbal tea include: controlling fever, boosting immune function, reducing inflammation, soothing the respiratory tract, eliminating ear infections, stimulating circulation, and easing constipation.

Enzyme A protein that catalyzes, or speeds up a chemical reaction. Enzymes are essential to sustain life because most chemical reactions in biological cells would occur too slowly, or would lead to different products without enzymes. A malfunction (mutation, overproduction, underproduction or deletion) of a single critical enzyme can lead to severe disease.

Essential fatty acid Fatty acids are required in the human diet. This means they cannot be synthesized by the body from other fatty acids and must be obtained from food. They provide elasticity to arterial walls and help prevent hardening of the arteries. They were labeled "essential" when researchers found that the removal of fatty acids from the diet harmed the normal growth of children and animals.

Essential nutrients A term for nutrients needed for building and repair that cannot be manufactured by the body, and that therefore must be supplied in the diet. At present, there are about 42 known essential nutrients.

Evening Primrose Oil Has remarkably rich stores of gamma-linolenic acid, which converts into prostaglandins in the body to regulate various body functions. May help to relieve the discomfort of PMS, endometriosis, and fibrocystic breasts. It may also ease joint pain and swelling of rheumatoid arthritis, help prevent diabetes associated nerve damage, reduce the symptoms of eczema, and help treat and alleviate the symptoms of a host of other ailments. It may interfere with anti-epileptic drugs.

Fennel tea Benefits of the fennel herb include: aiding digestion, detoxification, boosting metabolism, reducing stomach cramps, reducing heartburn, easing morning sickness and bloating, and flushing the kidneys. Fennel is also helpful after chemotherapy and radiation.

Food additive Substances added to food to preserve it or improve its flavor and appearance. Some additives have been used for centuries, such as vinegar for pickling or salt for preserving bacon. With the advent of processed foods in the second half of the 20th century, many more additives have been introduced, especially those of artificial origins. Food additives can be divided into many categories, some are: anticaking agents, acidity regulators, bulking agents, food coloring, color retention agents, emulsifiers, flavors, flavor enhancers, flour treatment agents, humectants, preservatives, stabilizers, sweeteners, and thickeners.

Food irradiation The process of exposing food to ionizing radiation in order to disinfect, sterilize or preserve it. Like most technology involving ionizing radiation, it is the subject of controversy regarding its safety. It is often called cold pasteurization or electronic pasteurization.

FOS Fructooligosaccharide (FOS) is also sometimes called oligofructose and is used as artificial or alternative sweetener. FOS use emerged in the 1980s in response to consumer demand for healthier and calorie-reduced foods. It is extracted from fruits and vegetables like bananas, onions, garlic, asparagus, barley, wheat, and tomatoes. The Jerusalem artichoke has been found to have one of the highest concentrations of FOS. It stimulates growth of bifidobacteria, friendly bacteria, that naturally populate the gut, increasing their ability to benefit overall gastrointestinal tract (GI) health, especially proper digestion.

Free radical An atom or group of atoms that is highly chemically reactive because it has at least one unpaired electron. Because they join so readily with other compounds, free radicals can attack cells and cause much damage in the body. Free radicals form in heated fats and oils as a result of exposure to atmospheric radiation and environmental pollutants, among other reasons.

Gamma ray The energetic form of electromagnetic radiation produced by radioactivity or other nuclear or subatomic processes such as electron-positron annihilation. Gamma rays form the highest-energy end of the electromagnetic spectrum.

Genetically modified food A product derived in whole or in part from a genetically modified organism (GMO) such as a crop plant, animal or microbe such as yeast. Genetically modified foods have been available since the 1990s. The principal ingredients of GM foods currently available are derived from genetically modified soybean, maize, and canola. Some governments have a strong mutual disagreement over the labeling and traceability requirements for GMO food products. For example, the European Union and Japan require labeling and traceability, while regulatory agencies in the United States do not believe these requirements are necessary.

Germanium This trace element enriches the body's oxygen supply by increasing tissue oxygenation and being a potent antioxidant. Both of these properties contribute to its widespread beneficial effects upon many inter-related metabolic process in the body.

Ginger root It is officially recognized as a remedy for appetite loss, indigestion, and motion sickness. However, ginger has a proven ability to combat all forms of nausea and vomiting. It is also taken to loosen phlegm, relieve gas, and tighten the tissues. Oriental Medicine also employs ginger as a treatment for colds and shortness of breath.

Glycemic index A ranking system for carbohydrates based on their immediate effect on blood glucose levels. It compares carbohydrates gram for gram in individual foods, providing a numerical, evidence-based index of postprandial (post-meal) glycemia.

Gray The gray (symbol Gy) is the SI unit of absorbed dose. One gray is the absorption of one joule of radiation energy by one kilogram of matter. KGy is a kilogray; 10^3.

Green tea The secret of green tea lies in the fact that it is rich in catechin polyphenols, particularly Epigallocatechin gallate (EGCG). EGCG is a powerful antioxidant; besides inhibiting the growth of cancer cells, it kills cancer cells without harming healthy tissues. It has also been effective in lowering LDL cholesterol levels and inhibiting the abnormal formation of blood clots. The latter takes on added importance when you consider that thrombosis (the formation of abnormal blood clots) is the leading cause of heart attacks and stroke. Green tea is also reputed to be helpful against infection and impaired immune function.

Gut flora Also called intestinal bacteria. It is the bacteria that normally live in the digestive tract and perform a number of useful functions involving the digestion for their hosts. The average human body, consisting of about 10^{13} cells, has about 10 times that number in microorganisms in the gut. Bacterial cells make up most of the material in the colon and 60% of the mass of feces. Somewhere between 300 and 1,000 different species live in the gut, with most estimates at about 500. The bacteria performs a host of useful functions, such as fermenting unused material to provide energy, training the immune system, and preventing growth of harmful species.

Hawthorn berries Known as the "heart herb," hawthorn has been used medicinally for heart health. It contains choline, which is said to break down cholesterol in the blood stream from large fatty clumps that can block veins and arteries, into tiny particles that can be utilized by the body tissues (emulsifies fat). Hawthorn also has an effect on energy levels and on the body's ability to burn up calories quickly by boosting metabolism.

Hormone A chemical messenger from one cell (or group of cells) to another. The function of hormones is to serve as a signal to the target cells; the action of hormones is determined by the pattern of secretion and the signal transduction of the receiving tissue. Hormone actions vary widely, but can include stimulation or inhibition of growth, induction or suppression of apoptosis (programmed cell death), activation or inhibition of the immune system, regulating metabolism, and preparation for a new activity (e.g. fighting, fleeing, mating) or phase of life (e.g. puberty, caring for offspring, menopause). In many cases, one hormone may regulate the production and release of other hormones. Many of the responses to hormone signals can be described as serving to regulate the metabolic activity of an organ or tissue. Hormones also control the reproductive cycle of virtually all multicellular organisms.

Immune system The system of specialized cells and organs that protect an organism from outside biological influences. When the immune system is functioning properly it protects the body against bacteria and viral infections, destroying cancer cells and foreign substances. If the immune system weakens, its ability to defend the body also weakens, allowing pathogens, including viruses that cause common colds and flu, to grow and flourish in the body. The immune system also performs surveillance of tumor cells, and immune suppression has been reported to increase the risk of certain types of cancer.

Indigestion A condition that is frequently caused by eating too fast, especially by eating high-fat foods quickly. Symptoms include a pain or burning feeling in the upper portion of the stomach; nausea; feeling bloated; uncontrollable burping;

heartburn; and a bitter taste in the mouth from stomach acid coming into the esophagus.

Junk food This is a derogatory term used for any food that is identified to be unhealthy and has low or poor nutritional value. Examples of junk food may include fast food burgers, French fries, potato chips, cookies, candies, donuts, soft drinks, and most processed and artificially preserved foods. Junk food is popular because it is very cheap to manufacture, is convenient to consume and has a lot of flavor because of its typically high fat, sodium or sugar content. Its nutritional value is usually low in nutrients and high in empty calories. Junk food also usually contains numerous food additives, which are used to enhance flavor, adjust texture, alter color, and prevent spoilage. For this reason, many junk foods are convenient because they have a long shelf life. However, what most people don't know or choose to ignore, is that junk food is addictive and extremely harmful to health. Since junk food is high in bad fats, refined sugars, and certain toxic chemicals, it is the leading cause of obesity, tooth decay, and increasing cases of diabetes, heart disease, cancer, etc.

Kamut A type of wheat that is similar to durum wheat. It is ideal for people unable to digest gluten, although it is unsuitable for those with celiac disease.

Kefir A fermented milk drink.

Kelp This is any of a variety of large, brown seaweeds that grow underwater and on rocky shores. Kelps are found in cold waters throughout the world. The kelp that has the most importance is Ascophyllum Nodosum, which grows in the cold Canadian waters of the Atlantic Ocean. Kelps supply 60 minerals, 21 amino acids, and 12 vitamins that are necessary for a balanced diet.

Lecithin A mixture of phospholipids that is composed of fatty acids, glycerol, phosphorus, and choline or inositol. All living cell membranes are largely composed of lecithin.

Lemongrass tea Lemongrass is used for reducing fever, stomach cramps, and flatulence. It eases arthritis pain and is a general digestive aid. It is especially suited for digestive problems in children.

Linoleic acid An Omega-6 polyunsaturated fatty acid used in the biosynthesis of prostaglandins and cell membranes. It is found in vegetable oils, especially sunflower oil.

Linolenic acid An Omega-3 fatty acid that is essential for all mammals. A particularly rich food source is flaxseed. It is also found in various oils, namely mustard, flaxseed, canola, soybean, pumpkin seed, and walnut oil.

Malabsorption The state of impaired absorption of nutrients in the small intestine. It has many different potential causes. Specific causes lead to different patterns of malabsorption. It may involve fat and fat-soluble vitamins (A, D, E and K); it may also affect vitamin B12, folic acid, iron, protein, and carbohydrates. Diarrhea is often present clinically, although this may not be the immediate cause for seeing a physician.

Malnutrition A general term for the medical condition in a person caused by an unbalanced diet—either too little or too much food, or a diet missing one or more important nutrients. Most commonly, malnourished people either do not have enough calories in their diet, or are eating a diet that lacks protein, vitamins or trace minerals. Medical problems arising from malnutrition are commonly referred to as deficiency diseases.

Mercury poisoning The phenomenon of toxification by contact with mercury. Mercury is a bioaccumulative toxin that is easily absorbed through the skin, respiratory, and gastrointestinal tissues. Mercury attacks the central nervous system and endocrine system and adversely affects the mouth, gums, and teeth. High exposure over long periods of time will result in brain damage and ultimately death.

Monounsaturated fat Dietary fats with one double-bonded carbon in the molecule, while all of the others are single-bonded carbons. Monounsaturated fats are healthier than other dietary fats for cooking and eating. Although they have the same concentration of food energy, they may result in reduced blood cholesterol levels, which reduce the chance for heart disease. Monounsaturated fats are found in natural foods like nuts and avocados, and are the main component of olive oil (oleic acid).

Niacin Also known as vitamin B3, niacin is a water-soluble vitamin and plays essential roles in energy metabolism in the living cell. Even a mild deficiency slows down the metabolism, which in turn decreases cold tolerance and is a potential contributing factor towards obesity. Niacin is often prescribed to combat high blood pressure and has been used in treatment of schizophrenia and other mental illnesses by orthomolecular practitioners.

Obesity A condition where the natural energy reserve, stored in the fatty tissue of humans, is increased to the point where it may impair health. Obesity in wild animals is very rare, but it is common in domestic animals that may be overfed and under exercised. In humans, it is generally considered to be one of the leading causes of health problems.

Organic food In general, a food that is produced without the use of artificial pesticides, herbicides, hormones, and genetically modified organisms (GMOs). The term *organic* is increasingly associated with certified organic foods, which are produced and labeled according to strictly regulated standards. Certification is a matter of legislation, and commercial use of the word *organic*, outside of the certification framework, is illegal.

Pau d' Arco tea Made from the inner bark of the Tabeluia tree in the Brazilian rainforest. It helps kill certain disease-causing bacteria, viruses, and fungi, partially justifying the name given to this herbal remedy, "tajy"—meaning to have strength and vigor. It can intensify the effect of blood thinners.

pH Power of hydrogen is a measure of the activity of hydrogen ions in a solution and, therefore, its acidity or alkalinity.

Phytochemical Also known as phytonutrients. Any chemical or nutrient derived from a plant source. More specifically, compounds found in plants that are not required for normal functioning of the body but that nonetheless have a beneficial effect on health or an active role in the amelioration of disease. Phytochemicals promote the function of the immune system, act directly against bacteria and viruses, reduce inflammation, and are associated with the treatment and/or prevention of cancer, cardiovascular disease, and any other malady affecting the health or well-being of an individual.

Preservative A natural or synthetic chemical that is added to products such as foods and pharmaceuticals. Preservative food additives are often used alone, or in conjunction with other methods of food preservation.

Propolis Bee propolis has been used by traditional medicine for its claimed beneficial effect on human health. It shows powerful local and antifungal properties. It is also efficient in treating skin burns and has been used to stimulate the immune system.

Protein Any of many complex nitrogen-based organic compounds made up of different combinations of amino acids. Proteins are basic elements of all animal and vegetable tissues. Biological substances such as hormones and enzymes also are composed of proteins. The body makes the specific proteins it needs for growth, repair, and other functions from amino acids that are either extracted from dietary protein or manufactured from other amino acids.

Prozac Fluoxetine hydrochloride is an antidepressant drug used medically in the treatment of depression, obsessive-compulsive disorder, bulimia nervosa, premenstrual dysphoric disorder, and panic disorder. This drug is also used off-label to treat many other conditions, such as ADHD. It is sold under the brand names Prozac, Lovan (Australia), Fontex (Sweden), Foxetin (Argentina), Fluctin (Austria, Germany), as well as Prodep and Fludac (India). Fluoxetine is a selective serotonin reuptake inhibitor (SSRI) and is marketed in capsules containing 10-90 mg of active ingredient. Prozac is not recommended for children under 18 years old.

Psyllium husk A bulk-forming agent that causes the stool to be bulkier and to retain more water, as well as forming an emollient gel, making it easier for peristaltic action to move it along. Psyllium husk should be taken with plenty of water. Bulk-producing agents have the gentlest effects among laxatives and can be taken just for maintaining regular bowel movements.

Pulse Defined by the Food and Agricultural Organization of the United Nations (FAO) as annual leguminous crops yielding from one to 12 grains or seeds of variable size, shape, and color within a pod. Pulses are used for food and animal feed. The term "pulses" as defined by the FAO, is reserved for crops harvested for the dry grain and therefore excludes green beans and green peas, which are considered vegetable crops. Also excluded are crops which are mainly grown for oil extraction, like soybeans and peanuts, and crops which are used exclusively for sowing, like clovers and alfalfa.

Quinoa A grain that is highly appreciated for its nutritional value. The United Nations has classified it as a super crop for its very high protein content. Unlike wheat or rice (which is low in lysine), quinoa contains a balanced set of essential amino acids for humans, making an unusually complete foodstuff. This means it takes less quinoa protein to meet one's nutritional needs than wheat protein. Quinoa also contains Omega-3 fatty acids, which provide benefit to the heart.

Saturated fat A type of fat that contains triglycerides containing only saturated fatty acids. Saturated fatty acids have no double bonds between the carbon atoms of the fatty acid chain (hence, they are fully saturated with hydrogen atoms). Fat that occurs naturally in living matter such as animals and plants and that is used as food for human consumption contains a varying proportion of saturated and unsaturated fat. Foods that contain a high proportion of saturated fat are butter, ghee, suet, tallow, lard, coconut oil, cottonseed oil, palm oil, dairy products (especially cream and cheese), meat, as well as some prepared foods. Saturated fat is very high in most fast foods and junk foods and has been consistently linked with obesity and an increased rate of atherosclerosis and coronary heart disease.

Senna tea A caffeine-free herb that is used as a natural laxative. Senna usually works 6-12 hours after drinking the tea at bedtime.

Serotonin A neurotransmitter synthesized primarily in serotonergic neurons in the central nervous system. Serotonin is believed to play an important part of the biochemistry of depression, migraine, bipolar disorder, and anxiety. It is also believed to be influential on sexuality and appetite.

Siberian ginseng Famed as an energy tonic in China since ancient times, Siberian ginseng only gained recognition in the West in the 1950s. Healthy men and women taking the herb were found to better endure physical strain, resist disease, and perform tests of mental sharpness.

Simple carbohydrates A type of carbohydrate that, owing to its chemical structure, is rapidly digested and absorbed into the bloodstream.

Spelt An important wheat species in Europe from the Bronze Age to Roman times. Spelt contains about 62% carbohydrates, 8.8 fiber, 12% protein, and 2.7% fat, as well as dietary minerals and vitamins, including silica.

Spirulina A blue-green algae with a coil-like shape that is a very rich source of nutrition. In fact, it was a staple of the Aztec diet. Spirulina is 55-70% protein. It contains vitamins A, B1, B2, B3, B6, B12, C, D, E, K, folate, biotin, beta carotene, pantothenic acid, and inositol. It also contains the minerals calcium, manganese, iron, chromium, phosphorous, molybdenum, iodine, chloride, magnesium, sodium, zinc, potassium, selenium, germanium, copper, and baron. Spirulina further contains phycocyanin, chlorophyll, and carotenoids, as well as gamma linolenic acid, glycolipids, sulfolipids, and polysaccharides. In addition, spirulina contains 19 of the 22 amino acids.

Stevia Also called sweet leaf, it is a genus of a bout 150 species of herbs and shrubs belonging to the sunflower family. Stevia is native to subtropical and tropical South America and Central America. For centuries the Native Americans of Paraguay and Brazil used stevia as a sweetener and to treat conditions such as obesity, high blood pressure, and heartburn. Today, it is widely used as a sweetener in Japan and is available in the United States and Canada as a health food supplement, but is used in place of sugar or artificial sweeteners.

Teff A species of lovegrass native to northeastern Africa. It is similar to millet in nutrition and cooking, but the seed is much smaller. Teff is believed to have originated in Ethiopia between 4000 BC and 1000 BCE. It is adapted to environments ranging from drought stress to water logged soil conditions. Teff is a grain that has a high concentration of different nutrients. It has a high calcium content and contains high levels of phosphorous, iron, copper, barium, and thiamin. The iron in teff is easily absorbed by the body. It is believed to enhance the performance of elite sportspeople. Teff is also high in protein and is considered to have an excellent amino acid composition (including all eight essential amino acids for humans) and has lysine levels higher than wheat or barley. Because of this variety, it stimulates the flora of the large intestine. Teff is high in carbohydrates and fiber and contains no gluten.

Toxin A poison that impairs the health and functioning of the body.

Traditional Chinese Medicine Also known simply as Chinese Medicine, it is the name commonly given to a range of traditional medical practices used in China that have developed over the course of several thousand years of history. It is also regarded as an instance of Oriental medicine, a term which may include other traditional Asian medical systems such as Japanese, Korean, Tibetan, and Mongolian medicine. Chinese medicine principally employs a method of analysis and synthesis, inquiring on a macro-level into the internal systems of the human body and their mutual relationships with the internal and external environment in an attempt to gain an understanding of the fundamental laws which govern the functioning of the human organism. This understanding is applied to the treatment and preservation of disease and health maintenance. Traditional Chinese Medicine is rooted in a unique, comprehensive and systematic theoretical structure that includes the Theory of the Five Elements, the human body Meridian System, Yin-yang, and other systems. Treatment is conducted with reference to this philosophical framework.

Unsaturated fat A fatty acid in which there is one or more double bonds between carbon atoms of the fatty acid chain. Such fat molecules are monounsaturated if each contains one double bond, and polyunsaturated if each contain more than one. Hydrogenation converts unsaturated fats to saturated fats, while dehydrogenation accomplishes the reverse. Substituting saturated fats with unsaturated fats helps to lower levels of total cholesterol and LDL cholesterol in the blood. A good way to remember is that unsaturated fats are liquid at room temperature.

Valerian root An herb used for sleeplessness, nervousness, and tension due to overwork, stress, and fatigue.

Vitamin A It protects dark green, yellow, and orange vegetables and fruits from solar radiation damage, and is thought to play a similar role in the human body. Carrots, squash, broccoli, sweet potatoes, tomatoes, kale, collards, cantaloupe, peaches, and apricots are particularly rich sources of beta-carotene.

Vitamin B12 Helps maintain healthy nerve cells and red blood cells. It is also needed to help make DNA, the genetic material in all cells. Vitamin B12 is found in the protein in food. Hydrochloric acid in the stomach releases B12 from proteins in food during digestion. It is naturally found in animal foods including fish, meat, poultry, eggs, milk, and milk products.

Vitamin B6 A water-soluble vitamin that is needed for more than 100 enzymes involved in protein metabolism. It is also essential for red blood cell metabolism. Hemoglobin within red blood cells carries oxygen to tissues. The body needs vitamin B6 to make hemoglobin. Vitamin B6 helps increase the amount of oxygen carried by hemoglobin. A vitamin B6 deficiency can result in a form of anemia that is similar to iron deficiency anemia. Vitamin B6 also helps maintain the blood glucose (sugar) within a normal range, and the nervous and immune system needs vitamin B6 to function efficiently. Foods rich in vitamin B6 include beans, meat, poultry, fish, and some fruits and vegetables.

Vitamin C A water-soluble compound that fulfills several roles in living systems. Important sources include citrus fruits, green peppers, broccoli, green leafy vegetables, strawberries, raw cabbage, and tomatoes.

Vitamin E A fat-soluble compound that protects lipids. Sources include wheat germ, nuts, seeds, whole grains, green leafy vegetables, vegetable oil, and fish-liver oil.

Vitamin An organic molecule required by a living organism for proper health. An organism deprived of all sources of a particular vitamin will eventually suffer from disease symptoms specific to that vitamin. Vitamins can be classified as either water soluble, which means they dissolve easily in water, or fat soluble, which means they are absorbed through the intestinal tract with the help of lipids. The term "vitamin" does not encompass other essential nutrients such as dietary minerals, essential fatty acids, or essential amino acids, nor is it used for the large number of other nutrients that merely promote health, but are not strictly essential.

Wheatgrass juice Wheatgrass is a young plant; a relative of wheat. Fresh leaf buds of this plant can be crushed to create a juice or dried to make a powder; the unprocessed plant contains high levels of cellulose that makes it indigestible. It possesses chlorophyll, amino acids, minerals, vitamins, and enzymes. The chlorophyll molecule is similar in structure to hemoglobin, leading some to believe that wheatgrass helps blood flow, digestion, and general detoxification of the body.

* * *